Aging with a Disability

Aging with a Disability

What the Clinician Needs to Know

Edited by

Bryan J. Kemp, Ph.D.

Director, Rehabilitation Research and Training Center
  on Aging with a Disability
Rancho Los Amigos National Rehabilitation Center
Downey, California

and

Laura Mosqueda, M.D.

Director, Program in Geriatrics, University of California,
  Irvine
Orange, California

THE JOHNS HOPKINS UNIVERSITY PRESS
Baltimore & London

© 2004 The Johns Hopkins University Press
All rights reserved. Published 2004
Printed in the United States of America on acid-free paper
9 8 7 6 5 4 3 2 1

The Johns Hopkins University Press
2715 North Charles Street
Baltimore, Maryland 21218-4363
www.press.jhu.edu

Library of Congress Cataloging-in-Publication Data

Aging with a disability : what the clinician needs to know / edited by
Bryan J. Kemp and Laura Mosqueda.
    p. ; cm.
Includes bibliographical references and index.
    ISBN 0-8018-7816-0 (hardcover : alk. paper) — ISBN 0-8019-7817-9
(pbk. : alk. paper)
    1. Aged people with disabilities—Medical care.
[DNLM: 1. Disabled Persons—Aged. 2. Aging. 3. Chronic
Disease—rehabilitation—Aged. 4. Health Services for the Aged. 5.
Rehabilitation—methods—Aged. WB 320 A2679 2004] I. Kemp, Bryan. II.
Mosqueda, Laura Ann.
    RC952.5.A4835 2004
    618.97—dc21
2003010636

A catalog record for this book is available from the British Library.

To people near and dear to us who contributed their support, patience, and love for a very long time:

Derek, Deron, Damon, Debra, and Devon Kemp
Robert Mosqueda

and to the loving memory of Gabriel Nava

Contents

Part 5. *Future Directions*

Acknowledgments

First, we thank the many people who participated in the research studies that led to the knowledge this book is based on. Not only did people with disabilities donate their time at the Rehabilitation Research and Training Center at Rancho Los Amigos National Rehabilitation Center and at the University of California, Irvine (UCI), but hundreds of people across the country have participated in research in other locations, including Oakland, Atlanta, New York, and Chicago. Without their taking time to share their perspectives and experiences, this book would not have happened.

We thank the authors of the chapters in this text. They have provided valuable and insightful views on topics critical to understanding aging with a disability. We also thank the two prime sponsors of our work, the National Institute on Disability and Rehabilitation Research (NIDRR), Office of Special Education and Rehabilitative Services, U.S. Department of Education, Washington, D.C., and the Centers for Disease Control and Prevention (CDC). Support from NIDRR has been both financial and professional. The Institute has supported two Rehabilitation Research and Training Centers on aging and disability at Rancho Los Amigos and UCI for several years (grant numbers H133B980024 and H133B70011), and we hope that this book can be seen as an outcome of that support. CDC partially supported a conference that brought together many of the faculty who contributed to this book, although the contents of their chapters are solely the responsibility of the authors and do not necessarily represent the official views of Centers for Disease Control and Prevention (grant number R13/CCR918432-01). We sincerely support the concept that individuals who have a disability have disease prevention needs as great as, or maybe even greater than, those of the rest of the population.

We thank our staff who helped so much in the production of this book.

Janeth Velazquez and Veronica Mendez served as coordinators, typing, retyping, and correcting multiple versions of each chapter while keeping a sense of humor about it all. Becky Mendoza, our administrative assistant, proofread the texts, created many of the tables and figures, and kept everyone sane. Finally, we thank our editor at the Johns Hopkins University Press, Wendy Harris, for her patience and counseling through the long process of creating this book.

Contributors

Rodney H. Adkins, Ph.D., Co-director, Spinal Cord Injury Project,
Rancho Los Amigos National Rehabilitation Center, Downey, California

William Bauman, M.D., Director, Spinal Cord Damage Research Center,
Veterans' Administration Medical Center, Bronx, New York

Susanne Bruyère, Ph.D., Project Director, Rehabilitation Research and
Training Center for Economic Research on Employment Policy for People
with Disabilities, School of Industrial and Labor Relations, Cornell
University, Ithaca, New York

Tamar Heller, Ph.D., Director, Department of Disability and Human
Development, University of Illinois at Chicago, Chicago, Illinois

June Kailes, Disability Consultant, Playa Del Rey, California

James S. Krause, Ph.D., Director, Department of Rehabilitation Sciences,
College of Health Professions, Medical University of South Carolina,
Charleston, South Carolina

Kathleen Lankasky, B.A., Director, Healthy Women Program,
Community Resources for Independent Living, Hayward, California

MaryAnn McColl, Ph.D., Professor, School of Rehabilitation Therapy,
Queens University, Kingston, Ontario

Kevin Murphy, M.D., Medical Director, Duluth Clinic, Gillette Children's Hospital, Duluth, Minnesota

Jacquelin Perry, M.D., Co-chief, Polio Program, Rancho Los Amigos National Rehabilitation Center, Downey, California

Michelle Putnam, Ph.D., Assistant Professor, George Warren Brown School of Social Work, Washington University, St. Louis, Missouri

Nancy Somerville, B.A., Research Associate, Project Threshold, Rancho Los Amigos National Rehabilitation Center, Downey, California

Lilli Thompson, P.T., Training Director, Rehabilitation Research and Training Center on Aging with Spinal Cord Injury, Rancho Los Amigos National Rehabilitation Center, Downey, California

Fernando Torres-Gil, Ph.D., Associate Dean, School of Public Policy and Social Research, University of California, Los Angeles, Los Angeles, California

Robert Waters, M.D., Chief Medical Officer, Rancho Los Amigos National Rehabilitation Center, Downey, California

Dorothy Wilson, O.T.R., Research Investigator, Project Threshold, Rancho Los Amigos National Rehabilitation Center, Downey, California

Terry Winkler, M.D., President, Ozark Area Rehabilitation Services, Springfield, Missouri

Aging with a Disability

Introduction

Bryan J. Kemp, Ph.D., and Laura Mosqueda, M.D.

For most Americans, life expectancy increased 60 percent between 1900 and 2000, from an average of just forty-seven years to about seventy-seven years. Major improvements in public health, the advent and widespread availability of antibiotics, better medical care (primary and specialty), and improvements in medical technology all were major contributors to this trend. However, most people with disabling conditions such as Down syndrome or spinal cord injury did not participate in this increase. As recently as 1945, an able-bodied person could expect to live about fifty-five years, while a person with Down syndrome could expect to live only sixteen years and someone who sustained a spinal cord injury had a life expectancy of just two years following the injury. Fortunately, this disparity has been reduced.

Today, life expectancy for a person with a congenital disability or a disability acquired early in life (before age twenty-five) is reasonably good. People with Down syndrome commonly live into their sixties and beyond. People with spinal cord injury have a life expectancy about 85 percent of that of their able-bodied counterparts. A growing number of people with various kinds of impairments, including cerebral palsy, rheumatoid arthritis, spina bifida, polio, developmental disorders, and spinal cord injury, are reaching and surpassing middle age. In fact, an estimated 12 million people are in this category!

These 12 million are the first generation of people with early-onset disabilities to live into middle and late life. Consequently we knew very little about how they might age. However, information, in the form of both anecdotal stories and research data, has been accumulating over the past twenty years that gives us an idea of the nature of that aging. What has emerged is a picture of atypical aging: these people frequently undergo substantial and even profound changes in health and functioning in midlife. These changes were neither anticipated nor planned for in earlier generations. The usual practice in rehabilitation was to urge people to do all they could do and to push a little (or a lot) past normal limits to maximize their abilities. Professionals in rehabilitation paid little attention to the long-term consequences of disability or the issue of aging. Living in the community, getting a job, fitting in, and having relationships were where it was at.

The first group to notice that aging was not going well was the population with polio. In the 1970s and early 1980s, people who had had polio began to notice fatigue, pain, and new muscle weakness. This complex, in the absence of other explanatory conditions, became known as postpolio syndrome. It may affect as many as 75 percent of all people who had polio earlier in life. Typically this change would occur in the late forties or early fifties. People who were fully functional would develop new disabilities, and those who were moderately disabled would develop major disabilities. They would often have to retire early, cut back on activities, ask for more assistance, and use higher levels of assistive devices. This has played havoc with their well-being: it is difficult to face a decline in health and functioning after struggling for so long to attain them.

It is becoming clear that people with other kinds of impairment encounter a condition similar to postpolio syndrome. That is, people with a history of cerebral palsy, spinal cord injury, Down syndrome, and other conditions appear to develop later-life complications that neither they nor their rehabilitation professionals expected. For example, people with cerebral palsy develop inordinate rates of orthopedic problems and falls. Those with spinal cord injury develop a variety of medical complications twenty to twenty-five years after onset, including cardiovascular disease, osteoporosis, and impaired glucose metabolism, to name a few. About one-third of people with Down syndrome develop Alzheimer disease by the time they are in their fifties. All people with early-onset physical impairments are at high risk of functional changes and new pain, fatigue, and weakness strikingly like what has been reported in the literature on postpolio syndrome.

People with disabilities often experience age-related changes in function fifteen to twenty years earlier than their nondisabled peers. It often seems to happen to those who are most active and productive. It is not uncommon to see a person with a disability change from being completely independent at age forty to needing more help and having to reduce activities by age fifty-five. This has important implications for our approach to rehabilitation. Previously accepted principles and practices may need to change dramatically to help these people live long, healthy, high-quality lives. In fact, the field of rehabilitation has seen several eras of significant change over the past hundred years.

The first era, largely up to the advent of antibiotics and the improvements in health care that occurred between 1900 and 1945, focused on survival. The main concern was to help people with serious illnesses and injuries survive. Before then—for example, during the Civil War and World War I—as many people died from infectious complications as from the wounds themselves. If a person could just survive an injury, a surgery, or a disease, it was considered a good result. There was no organized rehabilitation, and what happened from then on was mostly up to the family and to charity.

The second era in rehabilitation began in earnest during the 1940s. As more people began to survive the effects of war, injury, and disease, efforts were begun to rehabilitate them into society and the community. Specialized rehabilitation hospitals, such as Stoke-Mandeville in England and the Rusk Institute in the United States, focused on the needs of people with disabilities. During this era, many of the rehabilitation disciplines, such as physical therapy, occupational therapy, and rehabilitation psychology, developed into the highly professional specialties they are today. Issues such as improving physical functioning, returning to work, and finding improved technological solutions to problems of mobility were addressed aggressively. The first nonwooden wheelchairs were developed. During the 1950s, 1960s, and beyond, great advances were made medically, technologically, and socially in the care, integration, and rights of people with disabilities. This era reached a pinnacle with the passage of the Americans with Disabilities Act in 1991.

The third era is the era of longevity, and it began in the 1970s. Large numbers of people with disabilities existing from early in life began to live into midlife and late life. Issues of survival were still present, because not everyone has equal access to care, and people with disabilities are about six times more at risk of other health problems than their nondisabled peers. However, long-term survival is increasingly likely for most people. Reaching maximal function through rehabilitation is also more common than not. But increasing life expectancies do not always mean a long high quality of life. Disability finally met up with aging, but it appears that they met far earlier in life than anyone had anticipated.

This new era requires us to reevaluate rehabilitation practices and philosophy. Instead of encouraging everyone with a disability to work as hard as possible to enter society and to be accepted like anyone else, the "use it or lose it" attitude, we need to help them and their families plan for the long run. A philosophy akin to "conserve it to preserve it" may be more appropriate to the findings of research today. The emphasis on achieving maximal function probably began around World War II, when a general sense of "you can overcome anything if you just try hard enough" was common. Since society did not openly accept people with disabilities, they were encouraged to fit in or to pass as not disabled. This meant working hard to learn to ambulate, to get a job, to have a family, and to be like everyone else. In a sense, these people needed to be like professional athletes, putting out maximal effort every day. Recognition and rewards have led this model of behavior to become a way of life for many. However, the philosophy probably has long-term negative consequences.

This book is meant to educate professionals and students about the new era in rehabilitation by presenting current research and practice that can help professionals assist their patients and clients. The primary audience is practitioners and graduate students in rehabilitation professions, including physical and occupational therapy, nursing, medicine, rehabilitation counseling, social work, gerontology, and psychology. A secondary audience may be people who have disabilities and their families.

Our goal is to influence rehabilitation practice by emphasizing the changes that happen to many people with disabilities as they grow older. A second consideration is to help practitioners, both present and future, to realize that aging begins in the twenties. Aging is not the same as being aged. People begin to age long before they notice the changes normally associated with being old. This means that the best time to influence how you will age is when you are young. Small changes early in life can have a major impact on later life. In the case of nondisabled people, consider the effect on health and longevity of smoking versus not smoking for forty years: the changes do not necessarily show up early, but they usually do show up. In the case of a person with a disability, parallel thinking applies. What are the long-term consequences for joints of continuing to walk despite pain if a person has cerebral palsy? How long should a person who has a disability plan on working? Who will provide the support that parents give children with disabilities after the parents are gone? What are the long-term consequences of playing sports if you have a disability? What long-term health risks should be screened for regularly?

This book is divided into five parts. The first part provides the perspective of people with disabilities and their families about aging with a disability. Part 2 is about biopsychosocial issues, such as health and quality of life, that affect anyone who is aging with a disability. Part 3 discusses treatment considerations that are especially important for rehabilitation professionals. Part 4 addresses particular impairments, such as spinal cord injury, polio, cerebral palsy, and developmental disabilities. Part 5 looks to the future, with chapters on methodological issues in the study of aging with a disability and on implications for health policy; the final two chapters present contrasting views on barriers to care from the perspectives of the provider and the person with a disability.

As you read about aging with a disability in textbooks and articles, remember that some of our most important education comes from the people we serve: people with disabilities and their families. Listen, observe, discover, and learn.

Part 1

The Consumer's Perspective

1

A Consumer's Perspective on Living with a Disability

How Change in Function Affects Daily Life

Kathleen Lankasky, B.A.

I was about thirty-five years old when I started to feel the signs of aging that I later learned were being brought on prematurely by my disability (cerebral palsy). The timing was ironic, because it coincided with my involvement as the principal investigator of one of the country's first studies of how disability affects the normal aging process. Little did I know how much this study would change the way we look at the adult who is aging with a disability, and how much the assignment would touch and change my own life.

At that point I was just beginning to feel the then mysterious changes in my body: increased tightness in shoulders and neck, pain in joints and muscles, gastrointestinal discomfort (acid reflux), menstrual irregularities, and bladder weakness, to name just a few. Through sharing these changes with my peers (the one hundred participants in my study), I became aware that I wasn't alone with these symptoms, that they weren't "all in my head." These physical and functional changes are similar to the symptoms being experienced by hundreds of thousands of people aging with disabilities. This newfound knowledge both relieved and frightened me. It was a relief to know that I wasn't alone, that these symptoms weren't just my own problem. But I was frightened because aging with a disability was an uncharted course. We are the first generation living long enough to need answers to tough questions that have never been posed before.

Over the course of the study, I interviewed participants with a wide range of functional limitations, from very few limitations to total dependence on personal attendants for all activities of daily living. What began to register with me was that it isn't the level of physical functioning that limits one's potential for successful living and aging, but rather one's level of self-esteem and self-empowerment. It also became clear, through our discussions, that this self-esteem is a direct extension of the level of expectation for our lives expressed by our families and close circle of support (e.g., doctors, teachers, and therapists) as we grow up.

My concerns over the unforeseen changes in my functioning were validated as I realized that my experiences of aging with a disability were shared by my peers. But it also became apparent to me, as my interviewing came to a close, that each of our personal reactions to aging is unique and a product of many forces—forces that start in early childhood and have repercussions, both positive and negative, that last a lifetime.

I believe that a successful approach to living and aging with a disability had its roots in my childhood. My immediate social environment as a child had a lifelong impact on my sense of self-worth. These feelings of self-worth ultimately determined my ability to successfully face the challenges that go hand in hand with aging with a disability.

The more I listened to my peers describe their personal experiences of growing up and then getting older, the more I realized the importance of adequate self-esteem in coping with a disability over a lifetime, and the more I privately blessed my own parents for the self-esteem they had helped me to develop. This sense of personal worth helped me to meet the challenges of being a child laughed at by my peers, of exclusion by my teenage schoolmates, of acceptance by my husband, and of the effects of aging.

Successful Aging Begins in Childhood

In my family's case, as is true of many others, the rigors of life with a disability began early. The type of physical therapy program that was proposed for me, as a nonambulatory preschooler with quadriplegic cerebral palsy, involved six hours of hands-on physical therapy exercises (patterning) at home each day. My mother would spend most of her daytime hours manipulating my limbs, holding me as I attempted to mimic walking, and working with me on prespeech techniques. My father would take over when he got home from work, while my mother cooked dinner. As you can well imagine, my little brother, with all his physical abilities intact, was left pretty much to his own devices. That is, until one day during a therapy visit my physical therapist very bluntly said (I'm sure she had been rehearsing just the right words to use!), "You are crippling that little boy with neglect more than your daughter is disabled." My mother was lucky that I had an extremely perceptive physical therapist who cared enough to see what was happening to my brother and was willing to speak up.

After a good cry because she was devastated to realize that she had been neglecting my brother, my mother approached the problem the way she approached every challenge — head-on and with extreme determination. From that day on, Mom found all kinds of ways to include my brother in my therapy routine. He would hold my hand as I improved my walking ability, and he would help me learn to relax while falling by pushing me (without getting in trouble!) onto a pile of blankets when I least expected it. Through this experience, my brother began to take pride in being part of my habilitation. We became fast friends and have been ever since. Unfortunately, this is not so in many cases where one sibling has a disability.

Another early gift that my parents were strong enough to bestow on me was independence and the freedom to make my own mistakes. Life is full of mistakes, and our experience in making mistakes and learning from them is how we grow and develop our positive sense of self-reliance and self-worth, one of the key tasks of childhood. Unfortunately, many times children with disabilities aren't allowed the experience of making mistakes — like falling and getting back up — because of their parents' fear for their physical well-being. It's hard for parents to let go of their children even when they have no physical or mental vulnerabilities. For parents of children with disabilities, it may be nearly impossible.

My parents knew that I needed to learn from a young age how to live in a world that was primarily built for people without disabilities. This included negotiating the block between my house and my elementary school (never-ending to my small fearful eyes), with its icy, uneven pavement in winter and its slippery, leaf-covered sidewalks in spring and fall. Every morning my mother would send me off with a confident smile and a cheerful, "Have a great day, honey." After I was out of sight she would shut the door and cry. Mom knew there was a very good possibility that she would be called by the school or by a concerned neighbor to come pick up her child, who was crying from having skinned her knees. Skinned knees are common when a little girl with very poor coordination tries to negotiate just one block of uneven concrete. It would have been much easier simply to walk me to school, but my mother knew that I must learn to deal with the bruises of life if I was ever to gain the self-confidence necessary to live successfully and independently.

My parents' most important gift was their innate ability to see the necessity of keeping the whole child at center stage. I was always made to feel that I was a complete child — not just the sum of my disabled parts. It is easy for helpful professionals to forget that a child with a disability is a child first. In their enthusiasm to help her walk, or use her hands, or speak so as to be understood, caring professionals may forget that the child's sense of self needs to be the ultimate focus. While I was trying to learn to walk and to talk and to do all those physical activities that the other kids did with such natural abandon, it was very hard to keep my ego intact and to remember that I was a worthy person no matter how poorly I could use my physical body.

Learning to get back up from those early childhood falls was one of the necessary steps toward developing a full and fulfilling life, as a professional woman and as a wife in a twenty-five-year marriage, with two children who are successfully off to college. I emphasize my current happy situation because many of my peers with disabilities don't have mates or children — not because they are physically unable but because, as I see it, they received the wrong messages as they were growing up. They were led to believe that these normal milestones of adult life were out of their reach, and unfortunately these messages are ingrained early and are hard to erase by adulthood. Given that so many adults aging with disabilities live their lives based on this early misguidance, it is no wonder that a large majority of them reported feelings of isolation and loneliness during their later years in our study. One example was a man in his late fifties who had lived for many years with only a companion dog. At the point during the interview when I asked about his social support, he pointed down at his dog and sadly said to me, "This dog will be the only thing on earth that will miss me when I die." He passed away a few years ago. I wonder how many people even knew. I didn't.

Somehow my parents were able to routinely reinforce this positive sense of my own worthiness during my adolescence. One example occurred when I turned thirteen. As we all know, teenagers base much of their self-esteem on their perceived acceptance by their peers. This, of course, includes wearing the right clothes. Back in the mid-1960s, the "right" shoes for teenage girls happened to be penny loafers. Well, unfortunately, I needed the extra support of orthopedic saddle oxfords to walk without fear of falling. One day I decided that the saddle oxfords just had to go; I could not be seen in them at school ever again! I decided to approach my mother with the idea of buying penny loafers, even though I didn't have much hope of winning the argument. Without a moment's hesitation, she agreed with my "suggestion" (pleading), and we went out and bought my first pair of "normal" shoes. My mother knew that her teenage daughter's ego was more in need of therapy than were her feet. I felt like a million dollars in those penny loafers and continued to wear them for a couple of years, until I grew up enough to realize that it was better to stay on my feet than to look like everybody else. I put the saddle oxfords back on and haven't had them off since, but it was my decision to do so, not my parents forcing me. Again, they were quietly reinforcing my sense of empowerment.

As I look back over my years in public school classrooms, I remember with the most respect and gratitude those teachers who made me perform to the same level of expectation they had for their other students. One of the teachers I resented the most was my high school physical education instructor. She made me participate in all the activities required of her other students. I tried every excuse imaginable to get out of these most embarrassing of situations (square dancing, tennis, track), but to no avail. I now know that her message to me was never to rely on my disability as an excuse for not challenging myself.

Early memories can stay with us all our lives and even become barriers to accessing appropriate health care as we grow into middle age. For example, most adults with early-onset disabilities spent countless hours in one doctor's office or another, mostly male doctors. We were physically handled and looked at more extensively than children without disabilities. Unfortunately, even under the best of circumstances, all this attention to a physical body that doesn't work very well, and that surely doesn't look like the bodies of the other kids in the neighborhood, can have long-lasting negative effects on the child's self-image.

One consequence of these experiences was brought to my attention during an interview during our study with a professional woman in her mid-thirties who had cerebral palsy. At unforeseen moments during her hour-long commute to work every day, her legs would begin to spasm uncontrollably, to the point where the control of her car was in question. She was, in fact, beginning to question her own safety behind the wheel and even to fear losing her job. As part of the study, we were sending all our participants for a functional analysis and medical workup to a local physician who specialized in cerebral palsy. In this woman's case, I was especially pleased that we could offer her this opportunity to be seen by an expert. Perhaps she could find an answer to her wayward legs and not have to give up the job she so loved. Her enthusiasm matched mine until I casually mentioned that the physician asked that all participants wear gym shorts for their exams. All of a sudden her expression changed. "I've changed my mind. I don't want the physical," was all she said. Puzzled by the mysterious change of heart, I asked why and reiterated the possible benefits of talking to a specialist about her particular problem. Her response was incongruous with her previous appearance of personal and professional self-assurance. She responded very quietly but very passionately: "Do you know how many times as a little girl I was paraded, wearing nothing but gym shorts, back and forth, in front of groups of male doctors? They watched my movements without an ounce of respect for what their analytical, impersonal stares were doing to me as a person. I promised myself that I would never wear gym shorts and be put on display in a medical setting again." No amount of coaxing on my part could change her mind. A thirty-year-old emotional wound was barring her from the help that might have given her back control of her legs and saved her livelihood.

I Didn't Know Aging Started So Early

Most of my childhood and adolescence were dominated by seeking to become as independent as possible. Children and teens with disabilities experience the same urge and urgency to become independent as do nondisabled teens. During this most vulnerable of times, persons with disabilities must face the added challenge of surmounting their physical limitations while trying to ignore (usually) overprotective families. Independence and self-esteem go intimately together if you have a disability.

I never realized how strong the correlation was between my level of independence, my physical abilities, and my sense of self-worth until about age forty, when practically overnight all the skills I had taken so many extra years to master were mysteriously taken away from me. The disease started with a funny tingling in my hands whenever I bent over, and it progressed, over a five-month period, to a total lack of normal feeling in my extremities. Every day I would lose a little more of that hard-won independence. I started having more and more difficulty holding my eating and writing utensils. I could no longer pick up things I dropped. Tying my shoes and doing up buttons became impossible. I had to abandon many of my beautiful clothes for outfits without buttons or snaps. My husband or my children would tie my shoes for the day before they left for work or school. Can you imagine the sheer terror that was taking over my every waking thought? And on top of the dysfunction, there was the pain, the constant energy-draining pain, in my hands and my feet and all over my body when the disease hit its peak. My neurologist assured me that my new condition had nothing to do with my cerebral palsy, even though he admitted that the two conditions were probably exacerbating each other. Five months and hundreds of tests after the first symptoms caught my attention, I was diagnosed with peripheral neuropathy, a degeneration of the myelin sheaths that surround the peripheral nerves. My neurologist couldn't pinpoint a cause (diabetes is the most common one) or give me a prognosis for recovery.

I had two choices: I could roll up in a ball and give in to the depression that was quickly starting to steal away my energy, my passion for life, and my sense of self-worth, or I could decide that if I had had the gumption to learn to walk, feed myself, and write once, I surely could do it again! Over the next two years, while my husband and children did much of the everyday chores that I could no longer do without making huge messes, my brain learned to work with and around all the new and confusing sensations that my nerves were sending it. I slowly relearned chores like tying my shoes without feeling the shoestrings, feeding myself using larger-handled utensils, and writing with easy-grip pens. (I am at this moment typing on the computer by rote without feeling the keys.)

Of course I have had to make extensive adjustments in my physical activities over these past years. But to be honest, the largest and most significant adjustment I have had to make was in the way I had been judging my own worth as a human being. Was I really only the sum of my physical abilities, or did my worth run deeper than that? I quickly saw that my family and friends still wanted to be around me even though I could no longer "do" everything I had thought was so central to their regard for me. Not only that, but I began to realize that I was giving them a special gift of feeling needed by the very person who had always been the one to take charge. I was beginning to be able to judge myself based on being a good human being instead of a good human doing.

Fortunately I had a physician who did not dismiss my symptoms as "all in my head" and who did a thorough workup. This is not always, or maybe not even typically, the case. One example was the recent death of a good friend and a fellow founder of the Breast Health Access for Women with Disabilities Project, based in Berkeley, California. In 1994 Sue (not her real name) had gone to her doctor complaining of enlarged glands under her arms. Her doctor quickly passed off the symptoms as enlarged muscles developed by propelling her manual wheelchair. (Sue had become paralyzed from the waist down several years before but had maintained her very active life and love of playing sports—from a wheelchair.) A whole year later, after demanding a more thorough examination of her "enlarged muscles," she was diagnosed with stage two breast cancer. Five years after what seemed to be a successful treatment of the cancer, it reappeared, and she died within a few months. The question remains for all her friends to ponder. Would she have died if she didn't have a disability? What would have been different during that initial visit to her doctor?

Through the years of growing older with a disability, I have many times felt left out of the health care decision making that was going on around me instead of with me. I am the primary expert when it comes to knowing what is different about my body and my functioning today compared with yesterday. I have incredibly valuable input to add to the corpus of information so much of my health care is based on. I'm just now beginning to feel valued by my health care providers. Is it my advanced years and knowledge that have finally turned their heads, or is it a subtle shift in their attitude about their place in my life and my well-being?

For centuries, health professionals have been seen as healers of disease and fixers of broken bodies. Adults aging with disabilities realize they are far beyond "fixing." We're not looking to our health care providers and therapists for a "cure." We simply want to partner with them in finding ways to maintain an optimal level of physical and emotional health as we age further than any generation before us has ever dreamed possible.

Looking to the Future

The popular adage "You're as young as you think" is not quite as comforting to me as it might be to my peers aging without disabilities. As much as I want to feel young, my body is constantly reminding me, at age forty-nine, that I have put it through the wringer. I see my future more as a series of psychological readjustments than as changes in my medical and physical well-being. Based on the speed with which my walking and balance have deteriorated over the past fifteen years, I must come to grips with the fact that I will probably need a mobility aide, such as a scooter or powered wheelchair, sometime in the not-too-distant future. Does this concern me because of a fear of not getting around the community as well? No, not really. Does it bother me psychologically? Yes, most definitely. How do I let go of a physical ability that has been so much a part of my self-image for almost five decades? How do I give up the social status that this society seems to assign to "standing straight and walking tall"?

Over the past few years, as my physical abilities have been threatened in new and frightening ways, I have come to realize that my need for a circle of support from friends and medical professionals has never been stronger. Little comments and small gestures of respectful empathy have been my anchor on this uncharted voyage called aging—a voyage complicated by extra challenges brought on by my disabilities. During one of our visits in the aftermath of the added diagnosis of peripheral neuropathy, my psychologist, whom I have been seeing for more than twenty years, gave me a compliment that will stay with me forever. I was saying that I looked for a greater meaning in each of my challenges, so that I could go on with renewed perspective and strength. He quietly wrote down my thoughts on a sheet of paper and shoved it in his pocket without a word, letting me know that my ideas and coping skills were worthy of remembering and sharing with others in need.

Another gesture of respect that I will never forget was bestowed on me during a recent visit with my podiatric surgeon. He had gathered the entire orthopedic staff to join him one day to analyze an unusual problem I was having during my recuperation after a bunionectomy. Because of my uneven walk, I was overusing my "good" foot and subsequently having pain as my other foot was healing. Half of the doctors stood at one end of the hall and the other half at the other as I walked back and forth between them for what seemed like hours. At first, bad memories from my childhood of those long walks in front of doctors flashed into my head. But they were quickly erased by words of sincere respect coming from both ends of the hallway. Comments such as "You've done an incredible job developing your walking" and "What's your secret?" permeated the hallway as I less and less self-consciously showed them my progress. These medical professionals, in a matter of moments, made me feel like a valued member of their problem-solving team rather than a medical problem to be analyzed at arm's length. How quickly and easily a few friendly comments and nods of approval can defuse a potentially uncomfortable situation.

After the onset of the peripheral neuropathy a few years ago, I was able to get myself to look at the bigger picture and to make sense out of and accept the loss of speed and precision in my walking. Over time, a new contentment with my much slower self came over me, as I realized how many beautiful things I was beginning to see in my environment because I had to linger to conserve my energy and to keep from falling. More and more I would see beauty that went unnoticed by those around me. These moments have become special gifts that my new slower-paced life has given me. I wouldn't trade them for the most agile of bodies!

2

Family Members' Perspective on Aging with a Disability

Bryan J. Kemp, Ph.D.

Increased life expectancy and the concomitant changes in the health and functioning of people with disabilities have important implications for the family. Compared with earlier eras, this means that the members will have longer to live as a family and enjoy each other's companionship. But it also means that family members may need to provide more assistance and even caregiving for long periods. Certainly there is a need for long-term planning for assistance, economic security, and housing. Additionally, family members may have to deal with emotional issues resulting from caregiving or loss as well the strain of dealing with their own aging. This chapter describes the experiences of family members as they face many of these issues. It interweaves some information from research studies, but usually just to highlight a point. The information was gathered from in-depth interviews with members of families who are dealing with aging. These families were drawn from larger samples and were selected either because the identified person with a disability was undergoing substantial health or functional changes or because the family members were sophisticated enough to anticipate future changes and needs. These are not a cross section of families dealing with disability. Rather, they are a select sample facing issues they had not thought about before. This chapter is not about the families' adjustments to having a member with a disability or about the psychosocial or economic consequences, both positive and problematic, of that situation. Numerous books have been written on those topics, and family members are well aware of such concerns. Instead, this chapter focuses on issues related to aging, how families cope with them, and possible ways to help.

A family can be thought of as a system of people united by blood or by choice for the psychosocial purpose of providing stability and growth for its members. Like any system, it has demands placed on it, and it has processes to help meet those demands. The principal demands of a family consist of the needs of the individual family members (needs for safety, security, acceptance, development, etc.). Its principal processes include the providing of resources, communication among its members, support, affection, and, in the case of children, guidance. Having a family member with a disability changes the family system to various degrees, depending on the demands placed on it and how well its principal processes work. When the demands placed on a family or on one of its members are too great or when important family processes break down (or were never there in the first place), then the principal outcomes of family life—stability and growth for its members—are not met. However, just the opposite is also true: when a family does provide those elements, it can greatly aid its members, including those who have a disability. A study by Kemp, Adams, and Campbell (1997) illustrates this point. People with polio, people with postpolio syndrome, and people with no disability were objectively assessed for depression and were asked to rate their families on supportiveness, communication, and affection. People with postpolio syndrome (PPS) who had high family functioning had no more depression than the nondisabled people. But people with PPS who had low-functioning families had twice the level of depression of the nondisabled people. Thus good family functioning contributed to better coping with PPS.

There are many types of families for whom the topic of aging with a disability is important. Some have a member who is currently aging with a disability. Some have a child with a disability and need to think about the future. Each kind of family has slightly different issues affecting it, even though they all will have to address aging. They include:

- parents of a child with a disability
- older parents of an adult child with a disability
- a married couple in which one partner has a disability
- a married couple with children where one adult has a disability
- a person with a disability living alone but with family nearby

The following excerpts from interviews will illustrate these kinds of families.

Concern Starts Early and Continues

Fifty years ago, life expectancy for a child with a severe disability (e.g., spinal cord injury, spina bifida, cerebral palsy, Down syndrome) was only a fraction of what it is today. In 1930 life expectancy for a person with Down syndrome was only nine years; today it is about sixty. In earlier eras, the family support system was in place for the rest of that child's life. Today, parents are becoming aware that their children, with nearly normal life expectancies, will outlive them. The children will face many challenges in midlife and beyond, and plans must be in place to help. One important issue is, Who will care for my child? One couple, parents of a seventeen-year-old girl with cerebral palsy, expressed it this way:

Several years ago our daughter belonged to a local Girl Scout troop. In addition to selling Girl Scout cookies door-to-door and at parents' offices, the girls gathered at a local grocery store on a cool, bright Saturday morning in the fall to sell the remaining cookies. While the girls sold their wares to the shoppers, we settled into the grocery's delicatessen, drank coffee, and watched the girls in action.

We noticed an older man, probably in his mid-seventies, who was working as a bagger and helping customers load packages into their cars. He couldn't help but walk past our daughter Sally each time he went in and out of the store. On one trip he simply acknowledged her by saying hello; then he stopped and bought a box of cookies. Subsequently, with each trip he encouraged the grocery customers to buy from the girls, and soon he became their best advocate and sales representative.

About noon, we went outside, said something to our daughter about lunch, and stepped aside. The old man came up to talk to us. "Is that your little girl?" We said yes, and he made several positive remarks about her involvement with the Scouts. Then he said, "I have a little girl who uses a wheelchair too." "How old is your little girl?" my wife asked. "She's forty-six," he said.

He then explained that it was getting harder for him and his wife to lift her in and out of the tub and the bed and to help her with the toilet. We shared a number of experiences and observations. He and his wife had decided to keep their daughter home at a time when most children her age were institutionalized. There were no community services then, and they had done the best they could to care for her in their home and carry on their own lives.

Our families had obviously traveled down the same path, and there was much unsaid that connected us. We acknowledged their difficulty in caring for their daughter, and then in a remarkable moment of candor he observed, "I hope we live one day longer than she does." My wife and I both looked down and nodded, acknowledging his pain and concern.

I suspect the power of this event is in the fact that many parents of children with the most severe disabilities see their own lives played out in some fashion like that of this old man. There is a sense that resources, time, money, and capacity will run out before the need diminishes. Perhaps these fears are irrational, perhaps something will work out, but parents of adult children with disabilities—those with the most severe and demanding needs—never see others as giving their children the same attention and consideration that they provide. Who, for example, will turn our children at night, and who will make certain their clothing is neat? Who will be sure that braces fit and the wheelchair battery is fully charged? Who will do each of the thousand things that are so much a part of our lives but that seem utterly foreign to others?

This vignette captures both the emotional and the practical concerns of families. How will care be provided when the key people who have given it for so long can no longer do so? Therapists and other health providers are in a position to guide these families by pointing out the need for long-term care planning and for starting early in life a program to minimize unnecessary age-related losses. Fortunately, more families with children who have severe disabilities are becoming sensitized to the long-term issues of aging, often before the child is even an adult. Once, we at the Rehabilitation Research and Training Center on Aging with a Disability were conducting a workshop at a pediatric symposium in the Midwest. A therapist described a case in which she, the family, and her patient, a seventeen-year-old girl with cerebral palsy, disagreed about what kind of wheelchair the girl should use when she went away to college the next fall. The therapist wanted the girl to walk around the campus even though it was large and somewhat hilly. The therapist adhered to the "use it or lose it" philosophy of rehabilitation. The father wanted the daughter to use a powered chair, even though she could walk, because he had heard about the long-term consequences of ambulation on people with cerebral palsy (most develop orthopedic problems in midlife). He adopted the "conserve it to preserve it" philosophy. The daughter was caught in the middle and, being an attractive young lady, did not want to appear more disabled than she needed to, as the powered chair would signify. After the workshop, the therapist was going to recommend she use the powered chair for moving around the campus and walk inside classrooms and at home.

Aging Individuals, Aging Families

If the person with a disability is getting older, then the other family members are too. Sooner or later, the nondisabled person reaches fifty, fifty-five, sixty, and seventy years of age. With that aging often come changes in the other family members' health and functioning. And since families provide most of the assistance to people aging with disabilities, this can affect them all. Simultaneous changes in the family system can set the stage for a high degree of stress, as the following stories illustrate.

> Fred had been minimally assisting his fifty-five-year-old wife for twenty-eight years. Mary had had polio at an early age but was pretty independent. She worked, she enjoyed the family, and they had a good social life together. About four years ago, she began to develop postpolio syndrome and started needing more help with activities. She couldn't do the shopping anymore because of fatigue, she retired for the same reason, and she eventually lost so much strength that she couldn't get into bed or go to the toilet alone. Fred, who is now sixty-three, had never kept himself in really good shape. He was overweight and seldom exercised. One day, while helping his wife onto the toilet, he strained his back. The pain was considerable, and he found he could not lift her without aggravating his back injury. They have no children to help them, so they decided to try to find some in-home help who could come to the house a few hours each day. Mary didn't like a stranger helping her, but Fred could do only so much. They argued over loss of independence, intrusion in their life, the cost of help, and whether they should move to an assisted living facility. With no children, they feel they must solve their problems by themselves. The demands on their small family unit are beginning to show in increased stress.

The next case illustrates the impact of typical aging problems on top of age-related changes in the disability.

Esther is seventy-eight and has been disabled with an incomplete spinal cord injury since 1961. She was able to drive and work in the church and help raise her two children. As she approached her seventy-fourth birthday, she began to forget people's names,, recent conversations, and where she put things. Her doctor described it as "just getting older," but when it got worse, a year later she consulted a neurologist. The neurologist diagnosed her as having early Alzheimer disease. Her husband reports, "It's just one damn thing after the next! I just take it as it comes." Nothing could have prevented Esther from getting Alzheimer disease, but that on top of a spinal cord injury is probably going to create severe caregiving difficulties and stress for her husband.

An Example of Positive Adaptation

Barbara had polio at age nine months, and it left her weak in both legs, but mostly on the left side. She wore a brace on the left leg and simply did what everybody did as she grew up in her small midwestern town. When the other kids went skating, she watched from the sidelines but felt she was part of things. When the kids went skiing, she strapped on skis too and used the fence to pull herself up the gentle slope to slide down. Barbara did not think she had a disability because there was nothing she couldn't or wouldn't participate in one way or another. In the tenth grade, her parents asked her what kind of career she wanted. Recognizing that she was a bright student, they suggested dentistry or medicine, and she immediately chose medicine.

She did not consider herself to have a disability until about age twenty, when one of her professors suggested she use a cane. She graduated from medical school and began her career as a physician. She was happy. Her career was going well, she was married and had children. Then her husband was killed in an accident, and at age forty-five she was left with two children to raise, ages seven and ten. Thankfully, her position allowed her some flexible hours, and she was able to hire extra help as she needed it. Her health remained good, but over the next ten years she gained about twenty pounds. When she approached age forty-eight, she noticed that her better leg was growing weaker, so she started to use crutches to get around the hospital where she worked. She also felt more tired at the end of the day. By age fifty, the symptoms of postpolio syndrome were becoming evident, and she consulted a well-known expert. It was time to try other ways of getting around and setting priorities. Barbara began to use a powered chair part of the time; it saved her energy, and she noticed the difference.

Barbara had wanted to work until she was about sixty-two because that was what most people were aiming for, and she enjoyed her career as a doctor. However, by age fifty-five she recognized that her energy was giving out, so she changed her mind and retired at age fifty-eight. She spent the last year of her work using the powered chair almost full time because without it she could not get up and down the halls well enough. Since she has retired she has made even more changes to make her life easier and more enjoyable. First, she bought a more powerful scooter and a van so she could get around more easily. She also found she needed to set further priorities. Often she could do only one or two activities a day, so she chose to focus on the ones that maintained her social life, since that gave her the most enjoyment and the highest quality of life per unit of energy expended. However, two major events set her back. She developed a series of medical illnesses, and her mother's Alzheimer disease worsened to the point that Barbara could not look after her adequately at home. She felt that her body was letting her down even further, and she was depressed because she couldn't help her mother more, since she had been one of the main contributors to Barbara's success in life. Barbara sought professional counseling about these issues and to help her make the transition to the next phase of her life. She also joined a postpolio support group, which helped her recognize that she was not alone. And she lined up more help from the neighbors and from her daughter, especially with the chores she could no longer do. Her children learned not to overdo the help, which would have made Barbara feel dependent when she needed help only with certain things. Even the grandchildren learned how much Grandma could do and what she couldn't do. The family served as a valuable support and a source of enjoyment. They included her in all their activities.

What lessons can we learn from Barbara's experiences? First, she recognized the changes in herself and sought professional help for the physical and emotional difficulties she faced. Second, she accepted and used increasing amounts of assistance, both equipment and personal aid. Third, her family was adaptive and helpful, supplying the right amount of help without depriving her of the independence she needed. Finally, Barbara knew how to set priorities and to economize on her energy so that it went mostly to the activities that brought her the highest quality of life. Her family was supportive, adaptive, communicative, and affectionate. As a system, the family worked well.

It's Not What I Expected

Most people who became disabled fifteen, twenty, or thirty years ago didn't concern themselves very much with the prospect of a change in health and function around midlife. They believed or were taught that after reaching their maximum function through rehabilitation they would stay at that same level. Little was known about midlife changes due to overuse or health problems. Hence most people worked as hard as they could to achieve maximum function and to keep it. Slogans like "use it or lose it" reflected this ideology. Likewise, their families didn't expect that things would change very much. Only recently has research shown that people who have a disability often do have changes in their functioning, often early in life. These changes present important challenges to both the individual and the family, as the next three examples show.

> Betty Jo is now fifty-six. At age nine she had bulbar polio. Her mother told her, then and continually over the years, that she was actually lucky. She had very little disability; she was told that she couldn't get worse. Two years ago, she began to develop voice changes, with diminished volume, as well as pain in her back and legs and prolonged fatigue. She is now very worried that she is developing postpolio syndrome and feels betrayed by people, especially her mother, who promised her it would never get worse. She thinks that if she had known what she knows now, she would have taken things a little easier over the years.

> Robert and his wife have been married for thirteen years. She had a disability when they were married, but they both thought it would remain stable. Recently she began to lose function. He says of his experience, "Now I have to clean the house, and I admit that cleaning the house and doing windows is not a skill I am good at."

> Mary and Bill have been married twenty-three years. Bill has an incomplete spinal cord injury that occurred when he was a teenager. He is now fifty-one. Mary says of her present life with Bill, "I didn't expect that we'd have to reduce our social life and the things we liked to do together quite so much.

Now that the kids are raised and gone, I thought we would be able to travel more, not less. However, Bill's endurance is really low and he tires about 4:00 p.m. each day. He needs to go to bed to rest, so I've had to take up some activities without him. I feel really guilty about that but I can't just stay home all the time."

Harriet says of Dan, who had polio as a child, "I love him very much; we've had a good marriage. We never had really high-paying jobs, we got married out of high school and didn't go to college. Together, we've had a good enough income to live comfortably. I didn't think he'd have to quit working. We never heard of these midlife complications. Looking back, working as a grocery clerk was not the best thing for him to do. I think it put too much strain on his hips. I am now the only breadwinner, and he stays home. I can't blame him, but he's only fifty-five, and I think I'll have to work until I'm seventy just so we can make ends meet."

Conflict, Stress, and Strain

Conflict and stress can occur in families for many reasons: because of differences between people or because of problems attributed to one of the individuals. In families in which one person has a disability, both kinds of stress can be high. Conflict between individuals is often the result of role changes. Sociologists describe social roles as positions people have in relation to each other. Each role has its expected behaviors, rewards, and responsibilities. Changing roles, particularly if not voluntarily, can cause conflict and stress. One of the major role changes affecting families with a member who is disabled involves becoming, to various extents, a caregiver. The more one becomes a caregiver, the less time one spends in other roles, such as spouse, lover, or child. The following example highlights this.

Jerry has had changes in function with her cerebral palsy so that she now needs more help than ever. She has a great deal of pain in her legs and tires easily. Robert, her husband, used to go on fishing trips for several days at a time, but now he feels he can't be away that long. Robert says, "Sometimes I get cabin fever because of the time I spend with her. There are times when I wish there was someone to come in and give me a break of only one or two days so I could do something I enjoy. Financially this is not possible, so I just go on."

Sherri writes of her seventy-two-year-old mother with polio: "I wish I could just be her daughter. My mom's behavior because of postpolio syndrome has been full of frustration over her limited capabilities. Very many times, she takes the initiative in doing housework and yardwork, without bothering to ask my brother or father or me if I happen to be visiting. This often leads to overworking the leg, resulting in horrible leg spasms. Many times I will tell her not to do the work and to simply ask my brother or dad, but she insists much of the work will not get done unless she does it herself. I believe it stems from impatience and definitely without thought of what will happen to her. Unfortunately, this leads to frustration between her and my father and brother. My mother also tends to overwork herself at work. For a while, she was working many hours of overtime, worried about not being able to make ends meet. Of course this has had an effect on her, causing her to take a day off from work here and there. We've talked about possibly cutting down on the days she goes to work, but she still doesn't believe enough money will be coming in to pay the bills.

It's been very difficult for my mom to deal with the condition. I constantly worry about her overworking herself and encourage her not to take on so much because all the work will eventually get done.

I believe she needs to be more patient and accept the fact that she's not able to accomplish all the work she wants. She understands the condition she has but consistently overworks herself. She needs to understand she is doing more harm than good."

These examples show that sometimes increased needs for assistance and interpersonal problems can build to the point that emotions run high in both the person with the disability and other family members. Common reactions to increasing dependence are to deny the extent of the changes or to feel like a burden to others. Neither reaction is helpful.

Issues of self-worth, partnership, and role reversal and concerns about the future are stimulated by the changes people may undergo when they age with a disability. How to help families deal with these issues is described in later sections.

Balancing Needs

Two common complaints among family members are that they don't feel comfortable expressing their true feelings and that their own needs are not being met. It's not easy to express negative emotions like anger and disappointment to someone who appears to be feeling worse than you are. It seems unfair or selfish. Sometimes family members try to manage their anger and sorrow by trying harder. Sometimes they keep their feelings to themselves but believe they can't win. As one person said, "I try never to show her my feelings."

Harriet feels sorry for her husband because he's losing ability, but she knows he will misinterpret it as pity, which he had to deal with from the public decades ago, so she doesn't want to revisit it. Instead, she finds herself talking to her husband as if he were a child, then catches herself when she sees that she is changing her role from spouse to parent.

Jim has been assisting his wife with various activities for years. She already had a disability when they were married. He did more of the shopping than most men, and they had worked out a good system of dividing chores. He considered their relationship pretty equal. Then, about age fifty-three, his wife began to have increasing pain in her back, arms, and hands as well as considerable weakness. At times the pain is extreme and the fatigue overwhelming. It doesn't bother Jim that he now has to do more of the chores, but their sex life has nearly disappeared, and they seldom go out for an evening. Jim recognizes how difficult things have become for his wife, but at fifty-four he feels that many of his needs are not being met.

Helping Families Cope with Change

Help for families who are dealing with aging-related issues can be divided into three kinds, depending on the degree of stress present and the needs of the individual members.

1. *Education.* All families need information about age-related changes in health and functioning and what to do about them. The typical content for a group presentation to families should include the following topics:

   - age-related problems affecting people with disabilities
   - functional changes affecting people aging with disabilities

- managing age-related pain, fatigue, and weakness: dos and don'ts
- maintaining employment and other important roles
- maintaining quality of life while aging with a disability
- balancing the needs of all family members
- resources available for dealing with age-related changes

2. *Counseling.* About half of families could benefit from group or individual counseling. The difference between counseling and education is threefold. Education provides people with information, whereas counseling gives them more opportunity to learn skills. Second, counseling often focuses on emotion instead of information. People come to counseling to learn more about their own feelings. Third, counseling often is aimed at helping people cope better with whatever stresses they have in their lives. The stresses and strains of dealing with age-related issues can grow until they affect daily life, interpersonal functioning, and personal happiness. In these cases something more than education is needed. Family members need a situation where they can achieve the following results:

- discover whether the feelings they are having are normal for the situation
- improve communication between people with nonjudgmental understanding of the other person's perspective
- learn how to solve problems better so that most (not necessarily all) of each person's needs get met
- support other families going through similar experiences
- Group counseling like this can be open-ended. That is, people can start at any time and continue for as long as needed.

3. *Psychotherapy.* When stress becomes so great that a family member becomes clinically depressed, physically sick, or not able to function effectively in daily life, individual psychotherapy is needed, and group counseling should be avoided unless the person can use it as an adjunct to therapy. Perhaps as many as 15 percent of family members could profit from psychotherapy. The essential components of psychotherapy for situations surrounding caregiving issues include:

- a careful assessment of the person's physical and psychological health status

- prescription of appropriate psychotropic medicine if acceptable to the person
- twelve to twenty sessions of psychotherapy over several months
- focus on correcting unhelpful ways of coping
- improving ways to meet one's own needs and improve quality of life

There is evidence that short-term psychotherapy is helpful to most people (Hubble, Duncan, and Millar, 2000).

Summary

Families play an essential role in the lives of people with disabilities, a role that extends across childhood and adulthood and into late life. The recent discovery that the health and functional status of a person with a disability stands a good chance of changing by age forty or fifty has major implications for the family. Adjustments in the amount of assistance provided, the balancing of roles and individuals' needs, and the potential stress of these changes can greatly affect how the family functions. Because families provide more than 75 percent of the care for people who have disabilities, how well the family functions can affect both that person and other family members. Providing assistance without changing to a "caregiver" role (instead of the role of wife, husband, child, or parent) is a common challenge. Another new challenge is to plan for the long-term assistance that individuals will need and to decide how to provide for their economic, practical and interpersonal support. Families will need help to deal with these and other issues. That help may take the form of education, counseling, or in the case of severe difficulties, psychotherapy.

REFERENCES

Hubble, M. A., Duncan, B. L., and Millar, S. D. 2000. *The heart and soul of change: What works in therapy.* Washington, D.C.: American Psychological Association.

Kemp, B. J., Adams, B. M., and Campbell, M. L. 1997. Depression and life satisfaction in aging polio survivors versus age-matched controls: Relation to post-polio syndrome, family functioning, and attitude toward disability. *Archives of Physical Medicine and Rehabilitation* 78:187–92.

Part 2

Biopsychosocial Issues

3

Physiological Changes and Secondary Conditions

Laura Mosqueda, M.D.

What is "normal aging"? This seemingly simple question belies a complicated and important topic. Normal aging encompasses those age-related changes that are expected and inevitable; changes that cause disease or inability to function are not a part of it. Understanding the features of normal aging is not just an academic exercise: we must distinguish "normal" from "abnormal" so that we can know which age-related changes ought to be accepted and which ought to be prevented or treated. For example, diabetes is *not* a normal change of aging, but a gradual increase in insulin resistance is. We may therefore see that older adults have slightly higher average blood sugars than their younger counterparts, that there is no functional consequence from this normal change, and that no action need be taken. Diabetes, however, is an abnormal, pathological process that leads to a multitude of adverse consequences; it may be preventable, and it is certainly treatable. It is not a normal change of aging (Meneilly and Tessier 2000).

Newborns have a fairly predictable physiology and functional capacity. If a baby is born without an impairment, as most babies are, we know what to expect and when to expect it as the child develops: growth rate, developmental milestones (smiling, walking, speaking), increase in bone density, increase in functional capacity, and so on. Even at the ages of two, twelve, and twenty-two years, we can predict the functional capacity of most people with a high degree of certainty. However, as we mature many influences come into play and cumulatively affect our aging: genetics, habits, nutrition, environmental exposures, injuries, exercise, relationships, personality, and attitudes are but a few of these influences. These accumulated changes, which often start at the molecular level, eventually affect organ systems and lead to a wide range of physical, psychological, and social consequences. Each person is affected to varying degrees and in diverse ways so that as we age the differences among individuals become larger.

To illustrate the point, let's look at two women, Sarah and Jenny, both fifty-eight years old. They both had healthy childhoods and each is now married and has three children. Sarah's parents are alive and well; her mother is eighty-four years old, and her father is eighty-eight. Sarah has exercised three to five times a week for most of her adult life. She is in a happy marriage, has several close friends, and has a good relationship with her three adult children. Jenny's mother died at age sixty-two from complications related to breast cancer, and her father died of a myocardial infarction at age sixty-nine. Jenny does not participate in any regular exercise program. She attributes her ability to maintain her ideal body weight to her smoking a pack of cigarettes a day for the past thirty-five years; in fact, she is afraid she will gain weight if she stops smoking. Although these two people had similar physical capacities while they were growing up, these capacities began to diverge quite dramatically as they matured. Genetic influences and lifestyle choices favor Sarah. Her cardiovascular reserve is only slightly less than it was twenty years ago. On the other hand, it is likely that Jenny already has had a steep decline in her cardiovascular reserve capacity even though she is asymptomatic at present. While both women have the same chronological age, their physiological capacities are quite different; and the older they get, the more different they will become. This increase in heterogeneity of function over time is a hallmark of aging. It means that the older people are, the greater the interindividual differences. Figure 3.1 illustrates this point.

Age-Related Changes

It is not normal to experience diseases such as osteoarthritis and dementia as we age, but these common ailments occur at a higher frequency as we grow older. Health care providers as well as their patients often misinterpret them as normal changes and then fail to intervene because you don't treat "normal" conditions, you just accept them. Table 3.1 lists common and normal

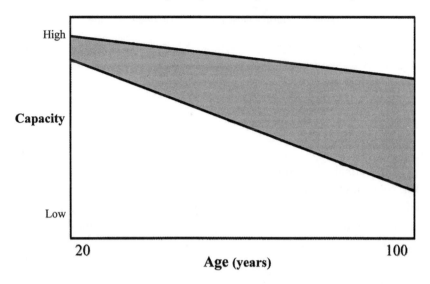

Figure 3.1. Heterogeneity in function increases with aging.

changes. This issue becomes more complicated when there is a preexisting disability. Because this is the first time in our history that large numbers of people with disabilities are living into middle age and beyond, we do not know what to expect and what to accept. Based on our understanding of normal aging, though, we ought not to accept new diseases and new disability as an inevitable consequence of aging with a disability.

At any point in time, there is a theoretical maximum level of physical function that each person has the potential to achieve. While few people actually attain this highest level, all of us have an upper limit that cannot be altered through activity, medication, or any other intervention. This level may be viewed from the perspective of each organ system (maximum capacity of the cardiovascular system, pulmonary system, renal system, etc.) or from the perspective of the whole organism (maximum ability to run, hike, ski, etc.). Most of us do not operate at or even near this maximum, nor is it necessary to do so. Olympic athletes are among the small percentage of people who push their bodies to their highest possible level of functioning. Perhaps people with disabilities share this characteristic with elite athletes; but instead of pushing their bodies to the limit during training in the quest for a gold medal, they must do so every day just to accomplish their daily activities and fulfill their social roles.

Table 3.1. Normal versus common changes with age

Normal	Common
Slower gait	Dementia
Gray hair	Depression
Lower bone density	Pain
Decline in renal function	Fatigue

With normal aging comes a gradual decrease in this maximum capacity. We know this intuitively: common sense tells us that a seventy-five-year-old athlete cannot beat a twenty-five-year-old in a hundred-yard dash even if they are both in the best possible condition. But why? The reason is the decrease in capacity that occurs over time. We must be careful to remember that this decrease does not in and of itself cause illness. It does, however, reduce the buffer zone we naturally have. This buffer zone, or physiological reserve, lets us cope with and recover from stressors. A decrease in physiological reserve occurs with normal aging. For example, a normal heart is capable of increasing cardiac output in response to vigorous exercise. With normal aging, one's heart rate still increases in response to exercise, but to a lesser extent; in other words, the heart's ability to respond to this increase in demand—its reserve capacity—diminishes.

All organ systems undergo a gradual decrease in reserve capacity, although at different rates for different people. In general, the decline in capacity is about 1 percent per year for most organ systems. For example, our creatinine clearance (a measure of renal function) goes down 1 percent per year after age thirty. Our pulmonary function undergoes a similar reduction in capacity. This rate of decline is influenced by genetics, lifestyle choices, and illness. People who smoke are likely to experience a more rapid decline in the physiological reserve of their pulmonary and cardiovascular systems than those who do not smoke. When there is no reserve capacity remaining, the organ system crosses a threshold into a state of disease. Buchner and Wagner (1982) define frailty as "the state of reduced physiologic reserve associated with increased susceptibility to disability." If an impairment occurs before age twenty to thirty (before one reaches one's peak physical/functional capacity), the maximum capacity may be reduced. A person who had childhood polio and required mechanical ventilation is unlikely to reach the same peak pulmonary capacity as a nondisabled counterpart. A person with cerebral palsy who has never

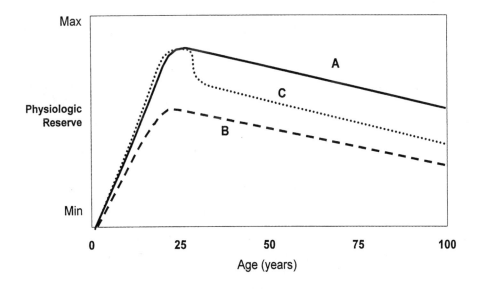

Figure 3.2. Example of decrease in physiological reserve: A, person without a disability; B, person born with a disability; C, person with a disability acquired at age thirty.

been ambulatory is unlikely to reach the same peak bone density as a young adult without a disability. These principles are described in figure 3.2.

The Baltimore Longitudinal Study of Aging (Shock et al. 1984) began in 1958. It was designed, among other things, to observe the changes in physiology that occur with aging. Initially only men were in the study, but women were included beginning in 1978. Clinical research evaluations occur every one to two years. This study reveals that most physiological functions show, on average, a gradual decline over the entire adult life. This is true of kidney, muscle, heart, lung, and nerve function: all show similar average changes with age. There is also tremendous variability among individuals in the rate of change (think about Sarah and Jenny), but this large data set shows us that when we are looking at populations the concept of decreasing physiological reserve is a reasonable generalization.

In *Successful Aging*, Rowe and Kahn (1998) used the concept of physiological reserve to make a distinction between "usual" aging and "successful" aging within the concept of normal (nonpathological) aging. Usual aging encompasses those who have little physiological reserve: they have no overt disease or disability but are at high risk for such. People who experience successful aging have a great amount of physiological reserve. They are described as having three critical behaviors or characteristics: low risk of disease and disability (which implies high physiological reserve), high mental and physical function, and active engagement with life. The book did not take into consideration people with early-onset disabilities. Experience shows us that those with long-standing disabilities are able to age successfully if they do not develop a new disability or functional decline (Whiteneck et al. 1992).

The Confluence of Aging and Disability

In her important book *Aging with a Disability*, Roberta Trieschmann (1987) asked: "Do many decades of living with a physical disability alter the aging process from what it would have been if the person did not have a physical impairment?" When she posed this question in 1987, there were few data that might provide an answer, but very many anecdotal reports gave a resounding yes!

The usual model of decreasing physiological reserve with age assumes there is no underlying impairment. What happens, then, when impairment and disability interact with aging? The answer partially depends on the age at which a disability is acquired. Let's think about two people, both with complete T-10 paraplegia, both of whom use a manual wheelchair, and both of whom are forty years old. One sustained a spinal cord injury when he was eight years old and the other did so at age thirty-eight. The amount of physiological reserve that each person has, despite their being the same chronological age, is quite different: the person who was injured at age eight did not develop the same degree of cardiovascular fitness or the same bone density as his counterpart. He has also used his arms to push a manual wheelchair for thirty more years than his counterpart, thus adding thirty more years of strain to his shoulders and wrists. When both experience the normal decline in physiological reserve that occurs with aging, the person who has been injured since age eight has almost no protective buffer zone and will likely develop osteoarthritis of the shoulders and carpal tunnel syndrome when he is only forty. The carpal tunnel syndrome may in turn lead to a series of complications: difficulty with mobility, transfers, and raises, pain, more medication, and even surgery with all its attendant risks. Thus, while chronological age is an important factor, it must be considered in the context of time since injury.

Physical Changes of Aging

It is important to have a working knowledge of normal age-related changes of the major organ systems in order to recognize pathology when it is present and to have realistic expectations for therapeutic interventions in middle-aged and older adults. One also needs some idea of how these normal changes interact with prior impairments and disabilities.

In the cardiovascular system, arterial walls become stiffer owing to changes in the properties of the elastin and deposit of calcium in the walls. This stiffening and narrowing is sometimes referred to as hardening of the arteries. As the arteries become narrower and less compliant, a higher pressure is required to perfuse the organs of the body. In fact, if blood pressure is maintained at too low a level with antihypertensive medications, this may itself damage the organs. Systolic blood pressures in the 140 to 160 range and diastolic blood pressures in the range of 80 to 90 are reasonable goals for people over age seventy-five.

Another normal age-related change is the decline of the maximum heart rate. This is particularly important during exercise or some illnesses, when an increase in cardiac output is needed (Ehsani 1987). Since cardiac output is the product of heart rate and stroke volume, the ventricles must dilate during exertion to accommodate the reduction in maximum heart rate. During exercise the heart rate may therefore not be a good indicator of strain on the person.

Total lung capacity does not change significantly with aging, but vital capacity, the largest breath a person can take, decreases. The functional residual capacity, the volume of air that remains in the lungs at the end of a quiet respiration, also increases with age. Each inhalation/exhalation cycle is a balance between the inspiratory muscles that expand the chest cavity and the elastic recoil of the lungs and chest wall that deflates it.

Older adults have a decrease in lung elastic recoil, which leads to compression of small airways during exhalation; this may in turn decrease arterial oxygen tension. While this loss of reserve does not cause a problem under normal (healthy) conditions, it may do so during acute illness, surgery, or—depending on the degree of physiological reserve—exercise. The diaphragm may weaken up to 25 percent with normal aging; this is not a problem unless a disease (such as pneumonia) puts an additional demand on the respiratory system.

Kyphoscoliosis, an abnormal curvature of the spine, is common in impairments such as cerebral palsy. Because the ribs originate at the vertebrae, the abnormal twists and turns of the vertebral column that occur with kyphoscoliosis distort the rib cage. This in turn distorts the size and shape of the lungs and impairs the muscles of respiration. As normal age-related changes combine with the effects of kyphoscoliosis, it is easy to understand why people with this condition may be at increased risk of pneumonia when they are only fifty.

Bone is a living, dynamic structure. It is constantly being broken down and reformed throughout our adult life. After age thirty there is a gradual decrease in bone density because formation of new bone does not keep up with the destruction of old bone. This decrease in bone density occurs in men and women at a rate of about 0.5 percent to 1 percent per year (see fig. 3.2). When women go through menopause there is a rapid reduction in bone density owing to a lack of estrogen. Of course, the greater their peak bone density, the more reserve they have at this time of rapid bone loss.

A common method of measuring bone density is dual-energy x-ray absorptiometry scanning. This noninvasive test uses radiation to estimate bone density. The two most common sites to be imaged are the vertebral column and the hips, both areas that are prone to fracture as we age. The data from the scan are compared with the average peak bone density of young people. By definition, "osteopenia" means the bone density is between 1 and 2.5 standard deviations below the norm for a thirty-five-year-old of the same gender. "Osteoporosis" describes a condition in which the bone density is more than 2.5 standard deviations below the norm. When a person has osteopenia or osteoporosis, the rate of bone resorption far exceeds the rate of bone formation, leading to a pathological state in which the bone fractures more easily. The relation between bone density and risk of fracture is dramatic: for every standard deviation decrease in bone mass, the fracture risk doubles (Ryan et al. 1992). This imbalance of resorption and formation primarily affects trabecular bone, the type of bone found in the wrists, hips, and vertebrae. Risk factors for osteoporosis include female gender, northern European origin, slender build, low calcium intake, loss of ovarian function, immobility, cigarette smoking, and excessive alcohol consumption.

Now consider a person who is born with a disability or acquires a disability at a young age. If she is unable to participate in weight-bearing exercise or has undergone periods of immobility (as often occurs, postoperatively, for example), she may never achieve the same peak bone density as her nondisabled peers; her physiological reserve of bone mass will be very small. When she then experiences the normal loss of bone mass after age thirty at a rate of at 0.5

to 1 percent per year, she may develop osteopenia or osteoporosis long before she reaches menopause.After a spinal cord injury, people undergo a period of rapid bone loss in the appendicular skeleton. One cross-sectional study found that people between ages twenty and thirty-nine with paraplegia or tetraplegia reach fracture threshold of the proximal femur in only one to nine years after the injury (Szollar et al. 1998). This finding translates into a high risk of fracture from minimal trauma (such as occurs with a transfer) for this cohort.

In their experience of caring for three hundred adults with cerebral palsy, a group of primary care physicians found a disproportionate number of adults with osteopenia (Rapp and Torres 2000). They postulated a variety of contributing causes: low calcium intake, infrequent exposure to sunlight (important in the metabolism of vitamin D), immobility, and use of medications (such as anticonvulsants) that decrease the ratio of bone formation to bone degradation. They also noted a worsening of bone density with age, as would be expected.

Osteoarthritis is common in people over sixty-five; for some people it is only a minor irritation, but for others it is quite disabling. This disease involves the degeneration of articular cartilage, accompanied by reactive changes in the surrounding area of the joint. Articular cartilage is normally composed of a few cells scattered within a matrix of collagen, proteoglycans, and water. This composition allows the cartilage to absorb the shock of weight-bearing exercise, thus protecting the underlying bone.

The causes of degeneration of cartilage are multiple, but experts agree that mechanical strain is one of them (Wise 2001). Imagine, then, a person who has been ambulatory his whole life despite significant lower extremity spasticity. The hip and knee joints were not designed to withstand the stresses placed on them with this gait, and he experiences the painful effects of osteoarthritis when he is only forty.

Many age-related changes occur in the skin. There is a decrease in the activity of the eccrine and apocrine glands, diminishing the ability to sweat. The epidermis thins, and the amount of subcutaneous fat decreases (although total body fat increases). The dermal and epidermal layers are closely interlocked in young skin; with aging there is a flattening at the junction so that much of the interdigitation is lost. Capillary walls become thinner with age and are more prone to rupture. Some of the consequences of these changes include delayed wound healing, impaired thermal regulation, increased propensity for skin to blister or tear, and increased susceptibility to bruising. These changes help explain why someone who has used a wheelchair since age twenty and has never had any skin problems starts experiencing skin break-down when he is only fifty. It also explains why it may take a long time for injuries such as pressure sores and lacerations to heal.

In young adults the kidneys filter blood through the glomeruli at a rate of 100 to 130 cc/min (the glomerular filtration rate). At about age thirty there begins a gradual decline in the glomerular filtration rate (GFR) that continues at about 1 percent per year. An estimate of renal function is reflected in the serum creatinine (Cr). Creatinine is a by-product of muscle breakdown. Because muscle mass decreases with aging, we might expect the serum creatinine to decrease as well. However, it happens that the normal decline in kidney function approximately parallels the normal decline in muscle mass, so that serum creatinine values remain relatively stable.

A more accurate reflection of the GFR is a measurement of the creatinine clearance, which can be estimated using the Cockcroft-Gault equation (1976). This equation takes into account age in years, ideal body weight (IBW) in kilograms, and serum creatinine:

$$CrCl = (140 - age) \; IBW/(72)(Cr)$$

For people with disabilities, it may be difficult to know the ideal body weight, since most tables are based on height and age. The ideal body weight for a forty-year-old, five-foot-two-inch woman with a C-6 spinal cord injury is probably not the same as the ideal body weight for a forty-year-old, five-foot-two-inch woman who is able-bodied.

This is not a trivial matter. Creatinine clearance has important implications for the many medications that are cleared by the kidneys. It is not uncommon for people with disabilities to have been on nephrotoxic medications, to have had frequent urinary tract infections (it's estimated that 30 percent of so-called simple urinary tract infections also result in silent infections of the kidney), or to have had long-standing renal disease. All of this contributes to the likelihood of adverse reactions to medications, which in turn increases the degree of disability.

Secondary, Associated, and Comorbid Conditions

As people with a disability age, a variety of new medical problems often arise. Some of these secondary conditions are a direct result of the primary impairment or disability. For example, people with spastic cerebral palsy are likely to develop contractures as they get older (Andersson and Mattson 2001). These contractures are directly related to the years of spasticity, which, despite diligence with range of motion exercises, eventually causes a fixed deformity. People with spinal cord injuries are more likely to develop pressure sores as they age (Johnson et al. 1998). Both of these examples of secondary conditions have potentially preventable components. Knowing this increased risk, the health care provider should educate consumers and should be vigilant in preventing or identifying these secondary conditions at the earliest possible stages.

Associated conditions occur with a higher frequency in people with certain impairments, although the direct link to the impairment is not obvious. For example, people with Down syndrome are much more likely than the general population to develop Alzheimer disease when they are middle-aged. This particular associated condition is understood to a limited extent: the same extra chromosome that results in Down syndrome contains a gene that is linked to an abnormal protein involved with Alzheimer disease. Another example is the link between spina bifida and latex allergies. This relationship is not so well understood, yet it is important that health care providers and consumers be aware of it.

Comorbid conditions are unrelated to the primary impairment and simply coexist with it. Parkinson disease, for example, is a common malady in the elderly. People with an impairment such as spinal cord injury or rheumatoid arthritis or postpolio syndrome are at neither increased nor decreased risk of this disease but may acquire it during their later years. While Parkinson disease is difficult enough on its own, a person with a preexisting disability will likely have a much harder time coping with this comorbid condition. As people with disabilities age, they are more likely to develop comorbid conditions. It is important to be aware of this because there may be a tendency, when a new problem arises, to attribute it to the primary disability, forgetting that this person may be experiencing a new, unrelated problem.

Summary

People who are aging with disabilities undergo numerous physiological changes that have a significant impact on their function. There is a tendency to accept these functional consequences as inevitable outcomes of aging. It is easy to be complacent and regard these changes as an unavoidable consequence of growing older. But as we gain a better understanding of what to accept, we also learn what not to accept; as we start anticipating changes (rather than waiting for them to occur), we also learn how to avoid some of the consequences that are common but not inevitable. As we get better at listening to our patients, we hear them tell us when subtle changes are occurring and know to take action. Good clinical skills, along with a solid understanding of the physiological changes described in this chapter, are fundamental to providing proper health care. We must also be willing to serve as educators and advocates so that we effectively translate our knowledge into actions that help our patients achieve a good, long life.

References

Andersson, C., and E. Mattson. 2001. Adults with cerebral palsy: A survey describing problems, needs, and resources, with special emphasis on locomotion. *Developmental Medicine and Child Neurology* 43:76–82.

Buchner, D. M., and Wagner, E. H. 1992. Preventing frail health. *Health Promotion and Disease Prevention* 8:17.

Cockcroft, D. W., and Gault, M. H. 1976. Prediction of creatinine clearance from serum creatinine. *Nephron* 16:31.

Ehsani, A. A. 1987. Cardiovascular adaptations to exercise training in the elderly. *Federation Procedures* 46:1840–43.

Johnson, R. L., Gerhart, K. A., McCray, J. Menconi, J. C., and Whiteneck, G. G. 1998. Secondary conditions following spinal cord injury in a population-based sample. *Spinal Cord* 36:45–50.

Meneilly, G. S., and Tessier, D. 2000. Diabetes in the elderly. In *Contemporary endocrinology of aging*, ed. J. E. Morley and L. Vanden Berg, 181-203. Totowa, N.J.: Humana Press.

Rapp, C. E., and Torres. M. M. 2000. The adult with cerebral palsy. *Archives of Family Medicine* 9 (5): 466–72.

Rowe, J. W., and Kahn, R. L. 1998. *Successful aging*. New York: Pantheon.

Ryan, P. J., Evans, P. , Gibson, T.. and Fogelman, I. 1992. Osteoporosis and chronic back pain: A study with single-photon emission computed tomography bone scintigraphy. *Journal of Bone Mineral Research* 7:1455–60.

Shock, N. W., Gruelich, R. C., Andres, R., Arenberg, D., Costa, P. T., Jr., Lakatta, E. G., and Tobin, J. D. 1984. *Normal human aging: The Baltimore Longitudinal Study of Aging*. NIH publication 84-2450. Washington, D.C.: U.S. Department of Health and Human Services.

Szollar, S. M., Martin, E. M. E., Sartoris, D. J.. Pathermore, J. G., and Deftos, L. J. 1998. Bone mineral density and indexes of bone metabolism in spinal cord injury. *American Journal of Physical Medicine and Rehabilitation* 77 (1): 28–35.

Trieschmann, R. B. 1987. *Aging with a disability*. New York: Demos.

Whiteneck, G. G., Charlifue, S. W., Frankel, H. L., Fraser, M. H., Gardner, B. P., and Silver, J. R. 1992. Mortality, morbidity, and psychosocial outcomes of persons spinal cord injured more than 20 years ago. *Paraplegia* 30:617–30.

Wise, C. 2001. *Osteoarthritis*. In *Scientific American medicine*, ed. D. C. Dale. New York: WebMD Professional Publishing.

4

Quality of Life, Coping, and Depression

Bryan J. Kemp, Ph.D.

Most people who have disabilities, whether congenital or acquired, want to achieve three things in life. First, they want (and need) to gain and maintain as good a health status as they can. In the case of acquired impairments such as a stroke, spinal cord injury, or arthritis, this means stabilizing whatever primary impairment caused the disability. And in all conditions (acquired and congenital) it means achieving and maintaining good overall health, the same as anyone else would. Second, individuals with disabilities want to improve their functional abilities as much as possible. These abilities include the fundamental underpinnings of all activity (strength, endurance, range of motion, and coordination) and extend to what are commonly referred to as activities of daily living (ADLs) and instrumental activities of daily living (IADLs) as well as employment, social, and leisure pursuits. Third, and most important for this chapter, they want to achieve a satisfactory quality of life (QOL). One expert even described high quality of life as the ultimate goal of rehabilitation (Crewe 1980). Quality of life means different things to different people, but it usually involves being able to participate in major life roles and having the kinds of experiences that make life worth living. Having a high quality of life also implies not being overwhelmed with feelings of distress or depression.

This chapter discusses recent findings pertaining to quality of life as a person lives with and ages with a disability. Fortunately, most people who have disabilities develop reasonably satisfying lives with good QOL. Unfortunately, many people find that new health problems and functional changes emerging in midlife threaten to erode the quality of life they achieved earlier. The issue of how to maintain a quality of life then becomes critical. It is therefore important for the treating health professional to understand what is meant by quality of life and what is known about what contributes to it.

The three outcomes that most people want from rehabilitation—health, functioning, and good quality of life—correspond to what the International Classification of Functioning, Disability and Health (World Health Organization 1993) labels *impairment* (health), *disability* (function), and *participation* (quality of life). Impairment is measured at the organ system level. The better the recovery from the primary condition, the less impaired the person will be. Likewise, the better a person can function, the less disability that person has in terms of being able to accomplish tasks, whether daily living tasks or employment. Participation is measured at the level of social integration. The greater the social integration, the more the participation. As we shall see, many of the factors that go into making a good-quality life exist on a social level and are intimately related to increasing participation.

The issues covered in this chapter are important for the treating therapist. It is vital to keep in mind the ultimate goal of most people with disabilities: to have as good a quality of life as possible. Being able to perform ADLs and IADLs is important and necessary, but they are seldom sufficient in themselves to promote a good-quality life. Therapists need to understand the activities and the roles that are important to their patients in developing and maintaining their quality of life, and they should help those facing mid- or late-life changes to preserve those activities as long as possible.

I begin with a review of what is meant by quality of life and the ways it has been measured, then present a conceptual model for understanding the factors involved in both positive QOL and negative QOL. Next I discuss the most common and serious manifestation of a negative QOL—depression—and the issues important to coping.

The Meaning and the Measurement of Quality of Life

Historically, two approaches have been taken to measuring QOL. One is objective, based on what are often called "social indicators"—factors such as education, housing, income, and employment status. The underlying assumption of this approach is that having more of these things makes for a better life and therefore a higher quality of life. Objective efforts to assess the quality of

American life began during the presidency of Dwight D. Eisenhower. A task force used several objective social indicators to assess the QOL of the country as a whole, including education, life expectancy, economic growth, health, and homeownership (Campbell, Converse, and Rodgers 1976). The results showed that the country had in fact achieved impressive gains since 1900. Life expectancy (at birth) increased from about fifty years in 1900 to about sixty-eight years by 1960. Homeownership increased from about 30 percent of the population to about 50 percent. Education increased to the point that most people had at least a high school education. It would be hard to disagree that quality of life improved a great deal for the country as a whole.

Objective measures of QOL also play an important role in assessing changes over time on these important social indicators and in comparing groups of individuals (such as people with disabilities versus nondisabled people) to see if equality exists. DeVivo and Richards (1992) used this method when they attempted to measure the objective quality of life of people with spinal cord injuries living in the United States. Using data from the National Spinal Cord Injury Statistical Center, they measured employment status, place of residence, education, and marital status after rehabilitation. By these standards, the quality of life of people with spinal cord injuries (SCI) was below that of the nondisabled population, and the results pointed to specific areas that needed improvement.

As important as objective indicators are, they often fail to capture how individuals feel about the quality of their own lives. Further, objective approaches also fail to sufficiently account for the fact that there is sometimes little correspondence between objective and subjective measures of QOL at the individual level. For example, a person who has a college education, a good income, and a home may still rate his or her QOL low, while a person with few possessions and little education may rate his or her subjective QOL high. The reason for this discrepancy is that most people evaluate their QOL based on their own perceptions, their expectations of how they think life should be, and what is important to them. Few people rate their quality of life solely by objective indicators.

The subjective approach to the measurement of QOL stresses individuals' appraisal of their own QOL. That is, QOL is high if people believe it is and low if they think so. Subjective approaches to the measurement of QOL use psychological scales to capture a perspective on these elements and to grade them. Sometimes an indirect measure of subjective QOL is used, such as life satisfaction, even though the terms are not synonymous. Research on subjective quality-of-life indicators achieved prominence with efforts centered at the University of Michigan in the 1970s. This research focused on the respondents' satisfaction with various parts of life, such as family, health, neighborhood, and friendships (Campbell, Converse, and Rodgers 1976; Flanagan 1979). Flanagan (1982) reported on quality-of-life research using the unique approach he called the "critical incident technique." This technique asks people to identify what they were doing when they last felt satisfied (the critical incident). Using this technique, he found there were fifteen factors, falling into five areas of life, that accounted for most of the satisfying feelings people had. The five areas were physical and material well-being, recreation, relations with other people, social and community activities, and personal development. Using this approach, he found, for example, that 90 percent of men in their fifties rated employment as critical for feeling satisfied, but far fewer men in their seventies rated employment as critical. Flanagan's work is important because it focused on what the person was doing that led to satisfaction.

Subjective measures of QOL also have their drawbacks. First, people may use different ideas of what is "excellent," "good," or "fair" in making their judgments. One person's "fair" is another person's "good." Second, ratings may be related to what people expect or what they've grown used to. This is especially relevant for those who have disabilities, because they may not have had ample opportunity to engage in social activities and thus may accept a lower objective level as "satisfactory" just because that's the way it's always been or the way they expect it to be.

Another problem is defining subjective quality of life. As Dijkers (1999) said, quality of life is a highly abstract concept, used by philosophers, economists, physicians, and psychologists alike to capture something about the value of one's life and the phenomenological experience of life. However, difficulties in measurement should not lead us to abandon the concept.

One approach to measuring QOL that has been used by the Rehabilitation Research and Training Center (RRTC) on Aging with a Disability at Rancho Los Amigos National Rehabilitation Center is described below. It uses a seven-point scale that involves placing QOL on a continuum from low to high. Figure 4.1 illustrates this model.

In the approach used by the RRTC, the participant is told: "Taking every-

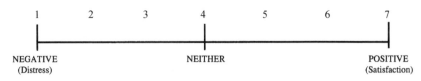

Figure 4.1. Quality-of-life continuum.

thing in your life into account right now, please rate your overall quality of life using this seven-point scale. (The person is shown the diagram.) Number 1 means 'Life is very distressing; it's hard to imagine how it could get much worse,' 4 means 'Life is so-so, neither good nor bad,' and 7 means 'Life is great; it's hard to imagine how it could get much better.'" The person then chooses a score, using half-point values if necessary, such as 4.5. This approach yields reliable results in the sense that when people are asked to repeat their ratings a week later, they are highly similar (Kemp and Ettelson 2001). Using this scale with over 700 people (500 with disabilities) indicated that scores from 1 to 4.5 are low (the bottom 25 percent of scores), scores of 5.0 to 5.5 are medium, and scores of 6 to 7 are high (the top 25 percent). Numerous questions can then be asked about the scores. For example: How do people with disabilities compare with able-bodied people? Which factors best describe people having low QOL versus high QOL? How do objective factors, such as severity of disability, relate to this subjective measure? And perhaps most important of all, if a person does have a disability, what factors relate to having a high quality of life versus a low quality of life? Figure 4.2 shows how many people with each type of impairment rated their QOL as high. These results show that on average, fewer people with disabilities rated their QOL high than did nondisabled people, and there were significant differences between groups.

Low Quality of Life and Depression

The low end of the quality-of-life continuum is characterized by feelings of unhappiness, isolation, and distress. The most typical way these experiences are manifested by people with disabilities is through the psychological disorder called depression. Numerous studies have shown that the combined prevalence of moderate and major depression is between 25 and 40 percent among people with disabilities who live in the community (Fuhrer et al. 1993;

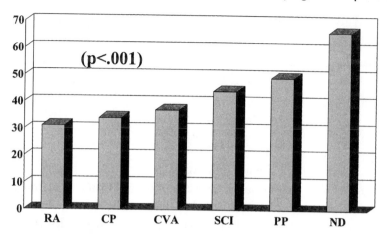

Figure 4.2. Percentage with high quality of life: RA, rheumatoid arthritis; CP, cerebral palsy; CVA, stroke; SCI, spinal cord injury; PP, postpolio syndrome; ND, nondisabled.

McColl and Rosenthal 1994; Kemp, Adams, and Campbell 1997). In other words, approximately one person in every three who has a disability also has either moderate or severe depression. This is about four times as high as among nondisabled people who live in the community. Besides the intense, distressing personal feelings that are part of depression, depression is disabling in itself and represents a serious and potentially life-threatening health condition. Depression causes increased disability, interpersonal problems, other health disorders, substance abuse, cognitive impairment, and loss of motivation. When added to a preexisting disability such as cerebral palsy or arthritis, depression may increase the level of disability by as much as 50 percent (Penninx et al. 1999). In a study of 1,300 people with spinal cord injuries, Krause, Kemp, and Coker (2000) found that rates of secondary health problems were three times higher in those who were depressed. Morris et al. (1993) found that the presence of depression reduced the chances of surviving for ten years by 50 percent for people with strokes. It is vital that therapists or other health professionals be able to recognize depression in people they assist and refer them for assistance if depression is suspected.

Depression is called a mood disorder because its primary symptom is a significant change in mood. The most common mood states associated with depression are sadness, irritability, and apathy. It is not necessary to be tearful or even sad to be depressed. Depression also causes symptoms in three other areas: physiological, cognitive, and behavioral. The core symptoms of depression are:

- a change in mood: a prolonged feeling of unhappiness, irritability, or apathy
- a change in physiology: altered sleep, decreased appetite, loss of energy, or loss of sexual function or an increase in pain, digestive problems, or fatigue
- a change in cognition: a diminished ability to concentrate, remember, make decisions or exercise reasonable judgment; thoughts of worthlessness, futility, death, hopelessness, failure, or guilt
- a change in behavior: decreased functioning in social roles or daily activities; a decrease in problem-solving ability and a decrease in pleasurable activities

These changes usually develop over the course of several weeks, eventually becoming severe enough to interfere with daily functioning or interpersonal relations, which then brings them to the attention of other people, such as family members or health professionals.

Symptoms of depression very often are overlooked or misidentified in people with disabilities because they often have significant health problems that are similar to the symptoms of depression. For example, pain, fatigue, poor sleep, and digestive trouble are common to both. Unless this overlap of symptoms is taken into account during assessment, people with disabilities may appear depressed when in fact they are not, producing a false alarm. More often, though, depression is missed for the same reason: symptoms that seem as if they are disability related (fatigue, pain, poor sleep, discouragement, difficulty with daily activities) are really due to depression. Several screening instruments have been developed to help identify people who may be depressed, and two of them are especially good for people with disabilities. Both are good for adults of any age, not just older adults: the Geriatric Depression Scale (Yesavage and Brink 1983) and the Older Adult Health and Mood Questionnaire(Kemp and Adams 1995). These are good for people who have disabilities because both scales minimize the physiological symptoms of depression, which can also be caused by the disability. Screening instruments like these can help to properly identify depression.

The Older Adult Health and Mood Questionnaire is reproduced in exhibit 4.1. It is a valid screening instrument for identifying adults who may be depressed. This scale was developed for use with adults who have disabilities. It was based on the criteria for depression described in the *Diagnostic and Statistical Manual* of the American Psychiatric Association (1994). Each of the odd-numbered items on the questionnaire relates to the mood disturbance associated with depression. The even-numbered items relate to the cognitive, behavioral, or physiological symptoms of depression. The score is the total number of "true" answers. Scores from 0 to 4 are considered normal, scores of 5 to 10 represent minor to moderate depression, and scores above 11 indicate possible major depression. The important point about identifying major depression is that treating it almost always requires medicine and psychotherapy, whereas moderate or mild depression usually responds to psychotherapy. As is true with all screening instruments, the results need to be followed up with an appropriate clinical assessment and medical evaluation to rule out other causes for high scores.

The Relation between QOL and Depression

It should come as little surprise that when depression is high, quality of life is low. In a study of 350 people with disabilities at the RRTC on Aging with a Disability, depression scores and QOL scores were collected. There were 185 people without depression, 113 with moderate depression, and 52 with major depression, making the overall percentage with a depressive disorder about 47 percent. For the group with major depression, the average QOL score was 3.1 out of 7. Only one person scored above 5 on QOL. In the group with moderate depression, the average QOL score was 4.9, with one-third of the group scoring below 4.0. However, in the group without significant depressive symptoms, the average QOL score was 5.9, and fewer than 10 percent scored below 5 on the QOL scale. In comparison, the average, score for 88 nondisabled, nondepressed people was 6.1, which was not statistically different from that for nondepressed people with disabilities. These results show two things: there is an inverse relation between QOL and depression, and in the absence of depression, QOL can be the same for disabled and nondisabled people. The high rate of depression among people with disabilities perhaps explains the lower QOL and life satisfaction scores often found in studies of them.

Exhibit 4.1. Older adult health and mood questionnaire

Directions: Decide if each question is mostly true or mostly false, then circle the correct answer.

1. My daily life is not interesting.	T	F
2. It is hard for me to get started on my daily chores and activities.	T	F
3. I have been more unhappy than usual for at least a month.	T	F
4. I have been sleeping poorly.	T	F
5. I gain little pleasure from anything.	T	F
6. I feel listless, tired, or fatigued a lot of the time.	T	F
7. I have felt sad, down in the dumps, or blue much of the time during the last month.	T	F
8. My memory or thinking is not as good as usual.	T	F
9. I have been more easily irritated or frustrated lately.	T	F
10. I feel worse in the morning than in the afternoon.	T	F
11. I have cried or felt like crying more than twice during the last month.	T	F
12. I am definitely slowed down compared to my usual way of feeling.	T	F
13. The things that used to make me happy don't do so anymore.	T	F
14. My appetite or digestion of food is worse than usual.	T	F
15. I frequently feel like I don't care about anything anymore.	T	F
16. Life is really not worth living most of the time.	T	F
17. My outlook is more gloomy than usual.	T	F
18. I have stopped several of my usual activities.	T	F
19. I cry or feel saddened more easily than a few months ago.	T	F
20. I feel pretty hopeless about improving my life.	T	F
21. I seem to have lost the ability to have any fun.	T	F
22. I have regrets about the past that I think about often.	T	F

Despite being higher among people who have disabilities, depression does not appear to be caused by disability in itself. This statement may seem surprising and even contradictory, given the results above. However, if depression were caused by the disability, then everyone with a disability would be depressed, and higher rates of depression would be observed among people who have more severe disabilities. Both assumptions are false. There is very little relation between rates of depression and either the severity of the impairment or the degree of disability. Several studies have shown the same result. For example, Fuhrer et al. (1993) assessed 100 people with spinal cord injuries who were living in the community. They found an overall rate of depression of about 40 percent, but there was no difference in the occurrence of depression between people with paraplegia and people with tetraplegia (quadriplegia). Similar results were reported by DeVivo and Richards (1992) and by Krause, Kemp, and Coker (2000) for other impairments besides spinal cord injury.

If depression is not caused by having a disability, then why is it more common among people who have disabilities than in people who do not? How do we account for the dual facts that (1) as a group, people who have disabilities have higher rates of depression than people without disabilities, but at the same time, (2) within groups of people with disabilities, there is little relation between rates of depression and severity of disability? Something appears to affect a lot of people who have disabilities, yet it is not associated with the severity of the disability. What could such a factor be? The answer appears to relate to stress and the way people differ in their ability to cope with stressful circumstances such as having a disability. Coping is itself a complicated topic; thousands of articles have been written about it. Perhaps the most widely adopted model of stress and coping is the one proposed by Lazarus and Folkman (1984) and elaborated on by others (Haley et al. 1996). This theory of stress and coping states that five important factors determine how much stress a person will experience in relation to life challenges: (1) the number and kind of life events a person has to cope with (particularly negative events), (2) the way the person appraises or interprets the meaning of these life events, (3) the social support the person receives in coping with negative life experiences, (4) the kind of coping methods the person actually uses to manage the emotional and practical aspects of the stressful events, and (5) the person's underlying and long-standing personality traits, such as being flexible versus rigid or optimistic versus pessimistic. Each of these variables interacts with the others to create a dynamic system of coping for each individual. For example, people with long-standing pessimistic personalities who are faced with adversity, such as the onset of a disability, will be prone to view the consequences in the worst possible way. Because of their sour outlook, they will not receive much support from others (who will get tired of the pessimism), and they will not select appropriate coping methods to combat the stress. The result will be a poor outcome. More optimistic people will not interpret events quite so negatively, will be better at eliciting support from others, and will use a greater variety of positive coping methods. The result will be a better outcome.

Using this model, we can postulate why people with disabilities have higher rates of depression than nondisabled people and, at the same time, why, within groups of people with disabilities there are no differences in depression between those who are more and less severely impaired. Of the five variables listed above, the one that is obviously most different between people who have disabilities and those who do not is the number of negative life events that occur because of their disabilities. With few exceptions, there is no evidence that most people who have disabilities start out having significantly different personalities, coping methods, appraisal systems, or social support systems than people who do not. However, people who have disabilities certainly have higher rates of medical, functional, social, environmental, and economic problems. Moreover, as other chapters in this book illustrate, even more negative life events may occur as a person ages. Therefore any impairment serious enough to cause permanent disability also creates an inordinate number of adverse life events. Coping with such a multitude of negative life events is difficult, and many people have trouble doing so. Thus, as a group, people who have disabilities have higher rates of distress and depression than people who do not. However, given that most people with disabilities have a higher number of negative life events, the other four factors then come into play to determine which ones will be most stressed. These factors do vary within groups of people who have disabilities, much the same as they vary among able-bodied people. And because these other variables do not appear to correlate with the severity of the impairment or the degree of disability, they become the important factors leading to the development of distress and depression. In short, the difference between groups is due to differences in the number of adverse life events, but the difference within groups is due to differences in appraisal, social support, coping method, and personality traits. Table 4.1 outlines these five important elements in coping and why they are important.

Table 4.1. The five factors involved in coping

Factor	Description	Why it's important
Life events	The number of negative life events, life changes, or losses per year is an indication of the potential stress a person is under.	In general, people can cope with two to four major stressors per year before it begins to exceed their capacity to cope and therefore places a strain on their coping resources.
Appraisal	Appraisal refers to the way a a person views or interprets the events in his/her life and the person's perception of the potential threat.	How people view the changes in their lives has been found to be as important as the changes themselves in determining the degree of stress that results.
Social support	Social support is how far a person feels emotionally supported and understood by others and helped by them.	Social support buffers the stress negative life events produce, and practical help reduces the number of tasks that must be done.
Coping method	The ways a person tries to reduce the stress constitute coping methods.	Some coping methods are better than others. In the long run, methods that try to avoid or emotionally escape stress are not as good as active or problem-solving methods.
Personality	Personality refers to a person's long-standing characteristic core traits, such as optimism versus pessimism, flexibility versus rigidity, and adaptability versus maladaptiveness.	Personality is a major factor in how a person will appraise events, the coping method that will be used, and the support that will be provided.

Studies show that as few as 10 percent of people in the general population who are depressed are adequately treated (e.g., Friedhoff 1994). Depression is even less likely to be treated among people with disabilities living in the community. There appear to be two reasons for this. First, depression is hard to detect in people who have disabilities, particularly if they have multiple medical complications. The symptoms of depression overlap with the symptoms caused by health problems and the disability. Both depression and disability can cause discouragement, fatigue, frustration, poor sleep, pain, difficulty starting daily activities, and worries about the future. Distinguishing when these are due to depression and when they are due to realistic disability-related health problems can be difficult for the average clinician. Second, even when depression is properly identified, clinicians often "normalize" it. In essence, clinicians often believe that if a person has a disability, it is "normal" to be depressed. And because "normal" conditions are not subject to treatment, the depressive disorder is not addressed. However, depression is never normal. Depression, particularly major depression, is an abnormal response to loss, change, and stress. While it is normal to become discouraged and frustrated or to become tired or lose motivation temporarily, those are different from becoming depressed.

Treatment of Depression

Depression is a treatable disorder, whether or not the person has an underlying disability. The most common types of treatment entail medication or psychotherapy or both. Modern medicines are generally safe, and refinements in psychotherapy techniques have made treatment more efficient. To determine the most appropriate form of treatment, several factors must be considered. First is the severity of the depression. Depressive disorders that involve many symptoms, symptoms that do not change with time or with support from others, or symptoms that greatly affect the person's functioning usually require both psychotherapy and antidepressant medication. The second factor is the person's cognitive status and ability to profit from verbal therapy. Most psychotherapy requires that a person be able to learn, to remember information after the therapy session ends, and to gain some degree of insight. People who are cognitively impaired can still benefit from psychological treatment, but their treatment may involve group socialization programs, activity therapy, and family education more than traditional psychotherapy. Third, it is important to understand the acute medical problems the person has, how these affect treatment (often by lengthening it), and how these medical conditions will influence which medicines a person can safely take.

The usual course of treatment that combines psychotherapy with an antidepressant medicine takes between six months and one year to complete. In the case of major depression, the first improvements are generally noted after about two to three weeks. The usual signs of improvement include a slightly improved mood, better sleep, a more optimistic outlook, and an increase in pleasurable activities. As treatment progresses we see further improvement in mood, increases in energy, better interpersonal relations, a more positive outlook, and better problem solving. Most people continue to take medicine for approximately one year. By then we hope that changes have occurred in their life or coping ability so that they can begin to taper off the medicine. Some people remain on medicine long term, usually because they have a history of recurring depression or because they become symptomatic when the medicine is withdrawn completely. Medicine is usually reduced slowly during the final phases of therapy, and most people return to their predepression levels of functioning. Approximately 80 percent of nondisabled people are substantially improved by treatment, making depression one of the most treatable of mental health problems.

One psychological issue seems prominent in the lives of people who are aging with disabilities as it pertains to the onset of depression. The many premature health and functional changes of the kind described elsewhere in this book often instigate depression. After a long period of improvement and stability and after having reached some level of maximum functioning and quality of life, people who experience premature age-related changes are often devastated emotionally to find that they now have to slow down, reduce or eliminate many of the activities they enjoyed, or spend more time dealing with health problems. These changes may occur much earlier than in nondisabled people, and this "out of life phase" change may initiate distress. For some people, the changes may signify that the disability has finally "won." They may have felt they had achieved a pretty normal life despite the disability, only to have premature losses come along and rob them of years of active life. The psychological challenge of maintaining a rewarding, meaningful, and productive life while combating the increases in health problems represents a major topic for psychotherapy. The issues are different than in learning to initially live with a disability. Now the person has to face issues of aging, but much earlier than he or she ever imagined.

Positive Quality of Life

In the proposed model of QOL, it was suggested that low QOL represents a state of distress that is often displayed as depression. However, the absence of such distress and low quality of life does not guarantee that a positive quality of life will follow. The absence of distress merely sets the stage for a more positive quality of life—it doesn't ensure it. The following section discusses findings about quality of life, the factors believed to be involved in positive quality of life, and how positive quality of life changes over the life span for people who have disabilities.

Research in this area, like research on other aspects of aging, has included both cross-sectional studies and longitudinal studies. In 1994 Lou Harris conducted a large cross-sectional opinion survey of the life satisfaction of people who have disabilities versus people without them. Those results showed that the overall life satisfaction of people with disabilities was slightly lower than the life satisfaction of people who had none. Areas that were particularly low were satisfaction with income and with health. Nancy Crewe and James Krause conducted some of the longest longitudinal studies of people with disabilities, specifically, people who had spinal cord injuries. In a series of articles (Krause and Crewe 1991; Krause 1992, 1997; Crewe 1996), they assessed and reassessed life satisfaction over a fifteen-year period. One of their basic questions was whether life satisfaction would remain stable or would change. Another issue was whether life satisfaction was more highly related to the age of the person or to how long the person had had a disability. This is important because if duration turned out to be the critical factor, it would suggest that experience living with a disability was the important variable. If age turned out to be the important variable, it would suggest that experience with life in general was the important factor in determining life satisfaction. They assessed life satisfaction on a scale with multiple subscales, including satisfaction with health, income, work, family, friends, and so on. They included people from age thirty to age sixty in their study and followed them for five, nine, eleven, and fifteen years. Although there were differences between subscales, the overall trend was quite clear. Life satisfaction scores increased to a maximum point at about age forty-five to fifty and then gradually began to decline. The areas that declined most were health and income, and the areas that decreased least were family and friends. These changes in life satisfaction correspond closely to what is known about the age of change in physical functioning for people who have disabilities. Studies of nondisabled individuals show that satisfaction with all these areas remains stable or even improves until a person is well into the seventies (Neugarten and Reed 1997). Thus the difference in length of time that life satisfaction will remain high for people with disabilities versus those without averages about fifteen to twenty years. These data were collected before much was known about the age-related changes in health and functioning that affect many people who have disabilities. The goal of future research and future clinical practice is to decrease the difference in life satisfaction between people with and without disabilities by discovering the underlying mechanisms and developing strategies to minimize the impact of aging on people who have disabilities.

In an attempt to further understand the factors involved in life satisfaction among people with disabilities, several investigators have examined which variables are most associated with it. Much of this research was summarized by two meta-analyses, one conducted by Dijkers (1999) and one by Fuhrer (1996). A meta-analysis is a way of summarizing a large number of research studies on the same topic. The procedure involves finding the average size of the relation between two or more variables across studies. This procedure provides stronger proof of the size of relations than any one study taken alone. Dijkers (1997) analyzed twenty-two studies that each included more than a hundred people. The combined samples had a very wide age range and a very wide distribution of times since onset (duration). This allowed him to examine whether age or duration was more important in relation to quality of life. In these studies, quality of life was measured mostly by life satisfaction scales. Also, each of the studies in the analysis included measures of impairment, disability, and social participation as defined by the World Health Organization. This approach allowed him to determine which of those three variables was most closely related to life satisfaction/quality of life. This determination is important because it helps to answer whether life satisfaction or quality of life is more strongly influenced by biomedical variables (like the severity of impairment), by the degree of functional limitations the person has (disability), or by the degree of social participation and community involvement.

In answer to the first question, he found that the average correlation between age and QOL was zero. Current age did not make a difference in life satisfaction. On the other hand, duration of impairment was significantly related to life satisfaction. The average correlation across studies was .21, meaning that the longer the duration of disability, the higher the life satisfaction score. This supports the idea that it is the length of time a person lives with a disability rather than just the number of years spent living that helps to determine life satisfaction. Dijkers then examined each of the components in the WHO model to determine which factors correlated most highly with life satisfaction. The average correlation between degree of impairment and life satisfaction was about .05, which is very weak. The correlation between disability measures and life satisfaction was about .20, which is moderate. But the correlation between various measures of social participation and life satisfaction averaged about .41, which is strong. When he further investigated which aspects of "handicap" were most predictive of life satisfaction, he found that formal social integration and social support were the strongest correlates. These results are important because they indicate that establishing a meaningful social life after incurring a disability is a key feature in creating life satisfaction and that life satisfaction can be high regardless of the severity of a person's disability.

How long does it take to reestablish life satisfaction and meaningful social integration after incurring a disability? If the results of the research by Krause and Crewe (1991) can be extrapolated, the time frame is about three to five years for adults. Putting things into perspective by comparing this with other outcomes, it seems that, notwithstanding complications, establishing initial control over the medical aspects of the impairment takes six months to a year, establishing maximum functional abilities takes one to three years, and reaching a meaningful level of life satisfaction can take three to five years. How long can a person with a disability then expect that life satisfaction will stay at its maximum before being at risk of declining? Here, results from Krause and Crewe (1991) suggest about twenty-five years' duration or forty-five years of age if the disability was acquired before age thirty. After then, life satisfaction could be challenged.

Research by Whiteneck et al. (1992) on people in England living long term with a disability suggests that this twenty-five-year time frame is likely. They studied people who had spinal cord injuries of at least twenty years' duration. Some of the people had experienced the kind of age-related changes described earlier in this book, and some had not. They then asked all the participants to estimate whether their overall quality of life was better currently or twenty years earlier. For people who had reported no changes in function, life currently was rated better than twenty years earlier. This is consistent with the notion that life satisfaction is associated with duration, everything else being constant. However, for those who had experienced substantial changes in their health and functioning, the period twenty years earlier was rated as superior. Thus, changes in function can have a dramatic effect on life satisfaction and quality of life.

In an effort to better understand the role of social and community activities on quality of life and to further develop a model of positive QOL, we at the Rehabilitation Research and Training Center on Aging with a Disability have investigated the role of community activities on quality of life. In a series of studies, the simple QOL scale described earlier was correlated with measures of community activities, activities of daily living, and instrumental activities of daily living. The working hypothesis was that QOL would be related to the number of community activities a person engages in and would not be strongly correlated with activities of a routine kind, such as ADLs and IADLs. The correlation between QOL and community activities was .40, while the correlation between QOL and ADLs was .13. The people with high QOL scores (6 and 7) averaged thirty-five community social interactions a week. The group with medium QOL scores averaged twenty-six interactions a week, and the group with low QOL (which involved many people who were depressed), averaged only fifteen interactions a week. Moreover, when QOL scores were compared between nondisabled and disabled participants, there was no significant difference as long as the groups were equated on depression scores and number of health problems.

What is there about community activities that makes them correlate more highly with QOL scores than ADLs and IADLs do? Perhaps community activities are more valued than ADLs or IADLs. Here we need to draw on the field of developmental psychology to help answer the question. We know that certain "themes" exist across the life span in terms of what motivates or satisfies people. In general, life can be divided into three phases: childhood, adulthood and late life. The theme of childhood/adolescence is pleasure. Children and adolescents are motivated to do things that feel good and that excite their senses. Children who end up depressed usually have more psychological and physical pain than pleasure in their lives. In adulthood, the theme of life becomes success and achievement. People want to get ahead and to achieve the signs of success. People in midlife who are depressed often report the opposite of success (failure) as an issue in their lives. Finally, in late life the theme becomes finding meaning and purpose in life. Their absence leads to despair and depression. Perhaps the reason community activities are correlated highly with QOL is that they provide a combination of pleasure, success, and meaning. Future research may further examine these issues. However, it is clear that quality of life does depend on being able to participate socially and to be active in the community.

Summary

Developing and maintaining a high quality of life is one of the most important goals for people with disabilities, whether the disability is congenital or acquired. A positive quality of life is more strongly related to social participation and length of time living with a disability than to the severity of the disability. Because people with disabilities often experience premature aging-related functional and health problems by middle age, the issue of how to maintain a positive QOL becomes important. For those who have a difficult time coping with such changes, depression often results. However, depression is a treatable disorder, and people with disabilities can be readily assisted. Help in maintaining a positive QOL means helping people to maintain community activities and important social relationships.

REFERENCES

Aaron, T., Beck, A., Rush, J., Shaw, B. F., and Emery, G. 1979. Cognitive therapy of depression. New York: Guilford Press.

American Psychiatric Association. 1994. Diagnostic and statistical manual of mental disorders, 4th ed. Washington, D.C.: American Psychiatric Press.

Campbell, A., Converse, P. E., and Rodgers, W. L. 1976. The quality of life of American life. New York: Russell Sage Foundation.

Crewe, N. M. 1980. Quality of life: The ultimate goal in rehabilitation. Minnesota Medicine, August, 586–89.

———. 1996. Gains and losses due to spinal cord injury: Views across 20 years. Topics in Spinal Cord Injury Rehabilitation 2:46–57.

DeVivo, M. J., and Richards, J. S. 1992. Community reintegration and quality of life following spinal cord injury. Paraplegia 30:108–12.

Dijkers, M. 1997. Quality of life: A meta-analysis of the effects of disablement components. Spinal Cord 35:829–40.

———. 1999. Correlates of life satisfaction in persons with spinal cord injury. Archives of Physical Medicine and Rehabilitation 80:867–76.

Flanagan, J. C. 1979. Identifying opportunities for improving the quality of life of older age groups. Palo Alto, Calif.: American Institutes for Research.

———. 1982. Measuring of quality of life: Current state of the art. Archives of Physical Medicine and Rehabilitation 63:56–79.

Friedhoff, A. J. 1994. Consensus development conference statement—diagnosis and treatment of depression in late life. In Diagnosis and treatment of depression in late life, ed. L. S. Schneider, C. F. Reynolds, B. D. Lebowitz, and A. J. Friedhoff, 493–551. Washington, D.C.: American Psychiatric Press.

Fuhrer, M. J. 1996. The subjective well-being of people with spinal cord injury: Relationships to impairment, disability and handicap. Topics in Spinal Cord Injury Rehabilitation 1:56–71.

Fuhrer, M. J., Rintala, D. H., Hart, K. A., Clearman, R., and Young, M. E. 1993. Depressive symptomatology among community-dwelling people with spinal cord injury. Archives of Physical Medicine and Rehabilitation 74:255–60.

Haley, W. E., Roth, D. L., Coleton, M. I., Ford, G. R., West, C. A. C., Collins, R. P., and Isobe, T. L. 1996. Appraisal, coping, and social support as mediators of well-being in black and Anglo family caregivers of patients with Alzheimer's disease. *Journal of Consulting and Clinical Psychology* 64:121–29.

Harris, L., and Associates. 1994. *NOD/Harris survey of Americans with disabilities*. New York: Lou Harris and Associates.

Kemp, B. J., and Adams, B. 1995. The Older Adult Health and Mood Questionnaire: A new measure of depression for older persons. *Journal of Gerontology Neurology and Psychology* 8:162–67.

Kemp, B. J., Adams, B. M., and Campbell, M. L. 1997. Depression and life satisfaction in aging polio survivors versus age-matched controls: Relation to post-polio syndrome, family functioning and attitude toward disability. *Archives of Physical Medicine and Rehabilitation* 78 (2):187–92.

Kemp, B. J., and Ettelson, D. 2001. Quality of life while living and aging with a spinal cord injury and other impairments. *Topics in Spinal Cord Injury Rehabilitation* 6 (3):116–27.

Krause, J. S. 1992. Longitudinal changes in adjustment after spinal cord injury: A 15-year study. *Archives of Physical Medicine and Rehabilitation* 73:564–68.

Krause, J. S. 1997. Adjustment after spinal cord injury: A 9-year longitudinal study. *Archives of Physical Medicine and Rehabilitation* 78:651–57.

Krause, J. S., and Crewe, N. M. 1991. Chronologic age, time since injury, and time of measurement: Effect on adjustment after spinal cord injury. *Archives of Physical Medicine and Rehabilitation* 72:91–100.

Krause, J. S., Kemp, B. J., and Coker, J. L. 2000. Depression after spinal cord injury: Relation to gender, ethnicity, aging and socioeconomic indicators. *Archives of Physical Medicine and Rehabilitation* 81:1099–1109.

Lazarus, R. S., and Folkman, S. 1984. *Stress appraisal and coping*. New York: Springer.

McColl, M. A., and Rosenthal, C. 1994. A model of resource needs of aging spinal cord injured men. *Paraplegia* 32:261–70.

Morris, P. L. P., Robinson, R. G., Andrzejewski, P., Samuels, J., and Price, T. R. 1993. Association of depression with 10-year poststroke mortality. *American Journal of Psychiatry* 150 (1):124–29.

Neugarten, B., and Reed, S. C. 1997. Social and psychological considerations. In *Geriatric medicine*, ed. C. Cassel, H. Cohen, E. B. Blasson, D. E. Meier, N. M. Resnick, L. Z. Ruberstein, and L. B. Sorenson. 3rd ed. New York: Springer.

Penninx, B. W. J. H., Leveille, S., Ferrucci, L., van Eijk, J. Th. M., and Jack, M. 1999. Exploring the effect of depression on physical disability: Longitudinal evidence from the established populations for epidomilogic studies of the elderly. *American Journal of Public Health* 89 (9):1346–52.

Whiteneck, G. G., Charlifue, S. W., Frankel, H. L., Fraser, M. H., Gardner, B. P., Gerhart, K. A., Krishman, K. R., Menter, R. R., Nuseibeh, I., Short, D. J, and Silver, J. R. 1992. Mortality, morbidity and psychosocial outcomes of persons spinal cord injured more than 20 years ago. *Paraplegia* 30:617–30.

World Health Organization. 1993. *International Classification of Impairment, Disabilities and Handicaps: Manual of classification relating to the consequences of disease*. Geneva: WHO.

Yesavage, J. A., and Brink, T. L. 1983. Development and validation of a geriatric depression screening scale: A preliminary report. *Journal of Psychiatric Research* 17:37–49.

5

Family and Caregiver Issues

Mary Ann McColl, Ph.D.

One of the issues facing people aging with disabilities is that their need for assistance with daily activities may increase as they get older. Even people who have placed a high value on their independence may find that as time goes by they need help from adaptive equipment or personal caregivers. Although there are only a few studies on the changing need for help and for adaptive equipment over time (Gerhart, Weitzenkamp, and Charlifue 1996), there is a "copious and diverse literature" dealing with caregiving in general (Kennedy, Walls, and Owens-Nicholson 1999).

This chapter offers some information on the changing need for help among people aging with disabilities. Because of the nature of the caregiving relationship, it is important to approach this task from two perspectives: the perspective of the recipient of care and the perspective of the caregiver. Thus the chapter will be divided into two main sections: the first draws on the literature as well as on research that offers firsthand insight into the changing need for care and assistance; the second section reviews the literature to elaborate the caregiver's perspective, including definitions of caregiving, profiles of caregivers, and factors affecting the perception of caregiver strain. The chapter concludes with a discussion of how both the care recipient's and the caregiver's perspectives are relevant for professionals working with people aging with disabilities.

The Perspective of the Care Recipient: The Need for More Help

The need for more help has been studied extensively in the elderly population and has become a particular concern for researchers as the number of older adults grows relative to the total population. In a large general population survey, Verbrugge, Rennert, and Madans (1997) found that functional difficulties in older people could be completely resolved in about 25 percent of cases with either personal or technological assistance. A further 50-60 percent of disability could be significantly reduced with assistance. They made an interesting distinction between personal and technological assistance. They found that personal assistance tended to be used for transferring and upper-extremity functions, whereas technological assistance, or equipment, tended to be used for problems involving the lower extremities or mobility.

From the perspective of care recipients, the main problems requiring assistance were with mobility and general activity level. Partridge, Johnston, and Morris (1996) found that the perception of overall health was closely tied to these two functions in a sample of older people living in the community, whereas specific health problems were not. Williamson and Fried (1996) also found that older people tended to attribute functional losses to "old age" rather than to any particular health problem, even ones that had been diagnosed. Thus, the need for assistance is closely tied to the perception of health.

To elaborate the perspective of the care recipient, the following results come from a study of 352 people from Canada, the United States, and England who are aging with spinal cord injuries. The findings are part of a longitudinal study in which individuals are interviewed every three years from twenty years postinjury onward. The sample consisted of 292 men (83 percent) and 60 women (17 percent), with an average age of 57.9 (± 10.6) and an average duration of disability of 33.7 years (± 8.2) (more information about the sample is given in table 5.1). Of these participants, 34 percent (113) reported that they needed more help than they had three years before, and 39 percent (138) reported a change in adaptive equipment in the past three years.

The most commonly cited reasons for these changes were age and illness, presumably leading to higher levels of disability. Pain and fatigue were also important factors that led participants to seek help. Interviewees also mentioned that gaining weight contributed to the loss of independence. Finally, subsequent injuries, such as fractures or soft tissue injuries, also led to changes in the need for assistance.

Those people who reported changing adaptive equipment in the past three years were most likely to have made a change to the wheelchair itself, although changes to transfer aids, cushions, and walking aids were also reported. About one-quarter of participants went from manual to powered chairs

Table 5.1. Details of the sample ($N = 352$)

	Frequency	Percentage
Age		
40–49	89	25.4
50–59	117	33.3
60–69	90	25.6
70–79	46	13.1
80+	9	2.5
Mean (s.d.)	57.9 (10.6)	
Gender		
Male	292	82.8
Female	60	17.2
Level of injury		
Cervical	143	44.1
Thoracic	150	46.3
Lumbosacral	31	9.6
Duration		
20–29	123	35.0
30–39	142	40.5
40–49	74	21.1
50+	12	3.4
Mean (s.d.)	33.7 (8.2)	
Completeness		
ASIA-A (5)	196	58.9
ASIA-B (4)	59	17.7
ASIA-C (3)	31	9.3
ASIA-D and E (2,1)	47	14.1

Note: There are some missing values that account for discrepancies in total N for different variables.

in the three-year window considered (table 5.2). An additional 27.6 percent acquired new wheelchairs, but this need not have accompanied a change in function; it may simply reflect the normal turnover of equipment. If we speculate that about half the population of aging wheelchair users changes wheelchairs every three years, then we conclude that, on average, a wheelchair lasts about six years.

A change in equipment and the need for more help are statistically correlated ($r = .125$; $p = .024$). These two variables are probably both associated with one of the factors mentioned above (illness, fatigue, pain, weight gain, etc.), and probably they are also associated with some form of contact with

Table 5.2. Changes in equipment
over the previous three years
(N = 136 cases)

	Frequency (%)	
New wheelchair	42	(27.6)
Powered chair	39	(25.7)
Transfer aids	29	(19.1)
Cushion	19	(12.5)
Hoist	15	(9.8)
Canes/braces	8	(5.2)
Total	152	

Table 5.3. Issues participants reported
needing more help with during the
past three years (N =113 cases)

	Frequency (%)	
Transfers	45	(34.1)
Housework	32	(24.2)
Dressing	11	(8.3)
Mobility	10	(7.5)
Everything	10	(7.5)
Toileting	9	(6.8)
Grooming	8	(6.1)
Reaching	4	(3.0)
Unspecified	3	(2.3)
Total	132	

professionals, who would be inclined to assess the effectiveness of existing equipment and to make suggestions about new products.

None of the other variables tested, including demographic, disability-related, or psychological variables, was significantly related to changes in equipment. Other than those changes brought about by a change in functional level, equipment changes often have to do with a number of nonsystematic factors, such as old equipment's wearing out or people's becoming aware of new options through friends or peers, advertisements, or trade publications.

With regard to increases in personal assistance, table 5.3 shows the functions people reported needing more help with. Less than 10 percent of the

Table 5.4. Differences between those who did and those who did not need more help in past three years

	Need more help (n = 113)		Don't need more help (n = 239)		p
Age	59.3	(1.0)	56.3	(0.7)	.012
YPI	35.3	(0.8)	32.5	(0.6)	.003
Level	8.1	(0.3)	7.9	(0.2)	n.s.
General health	7.8	(0.4)	8.8	(0.2)	.024
Disability problems (CPQ)	15.0	(0.5)	13.2	(0.4)	.005
Health problems (CPQ)	12.8	(0.4)	10.7	(0.3)	.000
Psychosocial problems (CPQ)	12.9	(0.5)	11.6	(0.3)	.024
Effects of fatigue	5.2	(0.6)	3.4	(0.3)	.010
Effects of pain	4.0	(0.6)	3.1	(0.3)	n.s.
QOL	2.7	(0.1)	3.1	(0.1)	.000
LSI	9.6	(0.5)	11.4	(0.3)	.002
CES-D	14.4	(l.1)	10.9	(0.7)	.003
Hours paid asst./day	3.0	(0.8)	2.2	(0.4)	n.s.
Hours unpaid / day	3.4	(0.7)	1.9	(0.3)	.037
Hours program / month	31.1	(10.6)	10.3	(1.0)	.053

YPI = years postinjury; Level = level of lesion (1 = C1,2, 2 = C3,4 . . . 13 = Sacral); General health = 1–10; CPQ = Current Problem Questionnaire (Krause and Crewe 1990); QOL (quality of life) = 1– 4; CES-D = Center for Epid. Studies—Depression (Radloff 1977); Effects of pain/fatigue = 7–35; LSI = Life Satisfaction Index (Neugarten, Havighurst, and Tobin 1961).

sample reported needing more help with everything; however, the most frequent issue was transfers—this affected 34 percent of the sample. Twenty-four percent needed more help with housework, and the other cases involved other ADLs (activities of daily living) such as dressing, grooming, and toileting. The focus on transfers may be because this is a relatively large category, including wheelchair, bed, toilet, bathtub, car, and any other transfers that are part of daily life. It may also be because of the enormous implications for overall mobility and independence associated with a loss of independence in transferring. Because of its centrality to independent functioning, even small changes in one's ability to transfer may be noticed and reported, because they have large implications.

Table 5.4 shows the results of a more detailed look at those members of our sample who needed more help. These 113 individuals were compared with the 239 who did not need more help, using t-tests and chi-square. Not surprisingly, those who needed more help were significantly older and had longer duration of disability than those who did not. They also reported poorer general health, more fatigue, and more of all three types of problems (disability-related, health-related, and psychological—using the Current Problem Questionnaire (Krause and Crewe 1990). Furthermore, they were significantly worse off on a number of psychological measures, including a four-point quality-of-life measure, a depression scale (the Centre for Epidemiological Studies Depression Scale, CES-D; Radloff 1977), and the Life Satisfaction Index (Neugarten, Havinghurst, and Tobin 1961). There was no difference in the need for assistance based on level of lesions or pain. In other words, people with higher lesions and people with pain were not more likely to have reported needing more help over the past three years when all other factors were taken into account.

With regard to the actual amount of help people required, we asked about three types: the number of hours per day of paid help (meaning out-of-pocket expenses); the number of hours per day of unpaid help (meaning informal caregiving, usually from family); and the number of hours per month of professional or programmatic help (covered by health insurance or government programs). Because there were three different countries, and therefore three different service delivery systems, this provided the best generic breakdown of service that was understood in all three countries.

Those people who reported needing more help received an average of 3 hours per day of paid help, which was not significantly different from those who did not report needing more help (2.2 hours). Thus, regardless of the perceived need for help, participants were paying for 2-3 hours of help per week, probably for housekeeping and other chores. They did, however, differ significantly on the amount of unpaid and program help required, with an average of 3.4 hours of informal caregiving per day and 31 hours per month of professional and other service. Assistance from these sources (family members or professional programs) is usually determined based on some external assessment of the need for help as well as the person's own assessment. Paid help, on the other hand, may depend on the ability to afford out-of-pocket costs rather than on the actual need for help.

Using logistic regression, a model was developed and tested to explain the need for more help. The model shows that the most significant predictor was an equipment change, underlining again that in many instances these two changes go together. We speculate that they both may accompany a precipitating event, such as a change in health status and the involvement of a professional, institution, or service. Those who changed equipment were twice as likely to need more help as those who did not.

Constipation was also a significant predictor of the need for more help, with those who experienced it having an 80 percent greater risk of dependence. This result is slightly more complicated to interpret, since it is unlikely that the need for more help relates directly to the bowel problem. Instead, this finding may signal the presence of other health problems, which may lead to inactivity and bed rest, which in turn may result in both constipation and the need for more help. Alternatively, constipation is a known side effect of a number of medications, particularly pain medications. Therefore it is possible that constipation again acts as an indicator of an underlying problem that causes both the constipation and greater dependence.

There was also a small increase in the probability of needing more help associated with the number of years postinjury. The odds ratio associated with years postinjury is 1.04, meaning that for each additional year of living with a spinal cord injury, there is a 4 percent increase in the need for help. At that rate, someone who lives twenty-five years with a spinal cord injury, as most people in our sample have, would have a probability of needing more help of 1.00. In other words, it is almost certain that they will begin to need more help beyond twenty-five years' duration. This is consistent with other literature showing a change is status at approximately thirty years' duration postinjury or fifty years of age (Krause 1992; Whiteneck et al. 1992).

Finally, life satisfaction had a small protective effect against needing more help. It is possible that being more satisfied with life leads one to be more independent. But a more likely explanation in a culture that values independence is that those who were more independent were more likely to be satisfied with life.

In summary, from the perspective of this sample of people living with disabilities:

- Age, illness or injury, pain, fatigue, and weight gain were all factors leading to the need for more help.
- Most of the issues people sought assistance with were basic ADL functions.
- People who needed more help reported more problems associated with health, disability, and psychological status.

- There was no difference in out-of-pocket costs for assistance but a significant difference in informal caregiving and programmatic help needed.
- Needing more help was related to a decrease in quality of life.

The Perspective of the Caregiver: The Determinants of Strain

From the perspective of the person providing the assistance, caregiving may be defined as taking responsibility for another person beyond those functions customarily associated with a defined role in a given culture (Schofield et al. 1997). A number of important ideas in this definition should be highlighted:

- Caregiving involves assuming a responsibility, usually one the care recipient previously took.
- Since responsibilities are typically associated with roles, taking on new responsibilities involves a change in role. Like all role changes, assuming caregiving functions needs to be balanced against other responsibilities and roles.
- Caregiving is part of a relationship, usually a family relationship. It often represents a new configuration of the relationship and may have pervasive implications for it.
- Caregiving functions exceed the normal expectations of a relationship. For example, when a wife provides personal care, such as assistance with bathing and dressing, this is considered caregiving. Despite promising in the marriage vows "to love and care for . . . in sickness and in health," husbands and wives in North American culture do not typically expect to assist one another with activities of daily living as part of the marital relationship.
- Caregiving can significantly affect the character of a relationship. Imagine a husband giving personal care to his wife or a son providing care to his father. Such an arrangement changes the fundamental balance between them and may affect other aspects of the relationship as well. The most obvious example of this is the change that may occur in an intimate relationship when the spouse takes on personal care functions.
- Finally, it is important to emphasize that the definition of caregiving

is culturally determined, and to be fully accurate we should refer not only to social and ethnic norms but also to family norms and expectations. Thus this definition of caregiving can be applied only in the context of an understanding of the cultural norms of each individual.

Another definition characterizes caregiving as a form of social support. The research is unequivocal that social support acts as a buffer against stress and thereby promotes recipients' health and well-being (McColl 1996). The primary caregiver is usually the most important source of instrumental support and often also of emotional support (Holicky and Charlifue 1999). Instrumental support refers to a broad category of social support that is practical or functional in nature and that can range from giving physical assistance with ADLs, to providing transportation, to lending money (McColl and Skinner 1992). In our research with people with spinal cord injuries (referred to earlier), we found that families provided 49 percent of the instrumental support that our sample received, 65 percent of the emotional support, and 41 percent of the informational support and guidance. Friends provided 32 percent of the instrumental support, 29 percent of the emotional support, and 26 percent of the informational support (McColl et al. 2001).

The number of caregivers in various countries has been estimated in national surveys, underscoring caregiving as a public policy issue. In 1992-93, a national survey in the United States estimated that 2.5 percent of the adult population provided care in the home for an elderly or disabled family member (Kennedy, Walls, and Owens-Nicholson et al. 1999). Of those, 89.5 percent were primary caregivers and 10.5 percent were secondary caregivers. That translates to more than 5 million Americans providing care in the home. In an earlier survey, Stone, Cafferata, and Sangl (1987) estimated that 2.2 million adults helped 1.6 million seniors with one or more of their activities of daily living. The difference between these two estimates is accounted for by the 40 percent of people with disabilities below age sixty-five, who were not included in the latter study. Australian estimates place the number of households where informal care is provided to a disabled member in the home at 5 percent (Schofield et al. 1997). These estimates compare closely with Canadian and British estimates (Howe, Schofield, and Hermann 1997).

The research shows us that caregivers are predominantly female (Schofield et al. 1997) and that they are typically the nearest female relative

(Kulkarni, Chamberlain, and Porritt 1992). Medeiros, Ferraz, and Quaresma (2000) describe the average caregiver as female, married, and forty years of age. This gender pattern is so evident that several authors characterize caregiving as an important issue in the study of women's health (Gaynor 1990; Bryant 1993).

Who Are Caregivers?

In terms of the relationship of the caregiver to the care recipient, there is agreement in the literature that there is a hierarchy of care providers, with immediate family at the top, then other relatives, friends and neighbors, and finally professionals. However, two large population-based surveys, one in America and one in Australia, disagree about who typically occupies the top spot. Kennedy, Walls, and Owens-Nicholson (1999), in their national survey in the United States, found that primary caregivers were most often spouses and were usually older and less healthy than secondary caregivers, who were usually daughters and in some cases sons. On the other hand, Schofield and associates (1997) in Australia found that 40 percent of caregivers were adult children, followed by spouses, parents, and others. Several studies have looked at the relationship of the caregiver to the care recipient in terms of caregiver effectiveness and strain and found that the closeness and quality of the relationship is the important determinant, not the fact that it is a wife, a mother, or a daughter (Coleman 1993; Schultz et al. 1994; Gillen et al. 1998).

Schofield and colleagues (1997) queried their sample about the amount of time they spent in giving care and the functions they performed. They found that approximately one-third fell into each of the following categories: less than 10 hours per week; 10 to 100 hours; more than 100 hours. Thus one might conclude that there are three categories of caregiving:

- minimal care, probably involving making appointments, organizing medications, minor ADL assistance of 1-2 hours per day;
- medium care, involving daytime supervision and some help with ADLs;
- heavy care, involving round-the-clock care and supervision.

These estimates of time commitment make it clear why for many people caregiving becomes an economic issue. For anyone providing either medium or heavy care, holding a job would be virtually impossible. A number of studies revealed that 15-20 percent of participants had given up their jobs to devote their time to caregiving (Liu 1991; Arnold and Case 1993; Schofield et al. 1997).

Caregiver Stress

Another important and consistent finding in the literature about caregivers is the high incidence of psychological disturbance: 22 percent of the spouses of stroke survivors were depressed (Bethoux et al. 1996); 47 percent of the mothers and spouses of brain injury survivors were depressed (Gillen et al. 1998) or troubled by anxiety (Novack et al. 1991); 37 percent of caregivers of people with rheumatoid arthritis had emotional disturbances (Medeiros et al. 2000). Thus it seems that, regardless of the origin of the disability, the caregiving function produces a psychological strain for a significant portion of the population.

In an effort to better understand caregiver strain and to counsel caregivers about ways to avoid strain, researchers have studied a number of factors thought to be related to negative psychological outcomes. The importance of this research lies in its ability not only to help caregivers themselves, but also indirectly to help care recipients, since psychological problems seriously inhibit caregivers' ability to provide effective care (Gallagher et al. 1994). The factors considered can be broadly classified into two categories: care recipient characteristics and caregiver characteristics. Care recipient characteristics obviously include the disability itself. Some authors have suggested that particular problems are more difficult for caregivers to deal with than others. For example, for aging caregivers, physical demands are obviously a source of strain. Bethoux and colleagues (1996) suggested that people were often sent home on the expectation of a certain level of functioning consistent with predischarge assessments. However, on returning home, this level of independence was not upheld, and within a short time people were demonstrating levels of dependency two to six times greater than they did in the hospital. This may be due in part to the willingness of spouses in particular to provide assistance. Schwartz and Kraft (1999) found that the more solicitous the caregiver, the more dependent the care recipient became. While the physical burden of caregiving on a spouse seems obvious, there is also a psychological burden associated with unmet expectations, disappointment, and frustration (Holicky 1996).

Another care recipient characteristic that caregivers consistently report finding stressful is a change in the essential nature of the individual or of the relationship. Behavioral, emotional, and cognitive changes, such as those incurred with Alzheimer disease, a stroke, or a brain injury, are particularly hard for caregivers to adjust to. Schofield et al. (1997) found that the most difficult behaviors for caregivers to cope with were memory problems, fatigue, diminished concentration, irritability, and confusion. In addition to these, Gillen and colleagues (1998) mentioned a lack of appropriate community services. These types of changes alter the basic relationship on which the caregiving commitment is made. The commitment to provide a particular level of care is based on certain beliefs about the relationship that was and that is or might be (Bethoux et al. 1996). Intrapersonal changes mean that this relationship is substantially altered, and caregivers may then feel they are devoting their time and a large measure of themselves to a virtual stranger.

One way this change in the relationship may be understood is in terms of the losses the caregiver experiences as a result of the onset or worsening of disability in a loved one. Mumma (2000) talked about three categories of loss: the loss of shared activities, the loss of the relationship, and the loss of one's own independence. Bethoux and associates (1996) referred to social, financial, and marital losses in their study of couples when one has had a stroke. Some participants had to move to a different home for accessibility or proximity to services; most experienced major changes in their social activities and contacts; many had out-of-pocket expenses that curbed spending on other things.

The actual number of problems experienced by care recipients is also an interesting determinant of the demands placed on caregivers. Logically, one would assume that more problems mean more care needed, with a potential for more strain or burden. Some studies have upheld this expectation (Coleman 1993; Semlyen, Summers, and Barnes 1998). However, a number of studies have shown that this is not the case. For example, our own work with people with spinal cord injuries in Canada and the United Kingdom showed that having more problems did not necessarily mean people received more help. Instead, having more support meant that they reported fewer problems, probably because some problems were dealt with by the caregiver (McColl et al. 2001). Thus the question arises whether the presence of problems acts as a deterrent or a stimulus to caregiving. One naturally hopes that caregivers respond positively to the obvious need for assistance; however, some literature suggests that the opposite is true: that the need for more assistance may frighten potential caregivers away (Periard 1989). Our research shows that neither is the case; support is not determined by the presence or absence of problems but instead depends on a host of other social and psychological factors.

The second category of factors affecting caregiver strain are characteristics of the caregivers themselves. Several studies found that the most significant predictor of psychological distress in caregivers is the prior existence of psychological problems. For example, Gillen and colleagues (1998) found very high levels of depression in their sample of mothers and spouses of people with brain injuries (43-47 percent). However, 70 percent of those diagnosed at time 1 had a diagnosis of depression before the onset of traumatic brain injury, and 65 percent of those diagnosed at time 2 had been positive at time 1. This finding emphasizes the need for attention to the psychological history of the caregiver in helping to identify those at risk of caregiver burn-out.

Along the same lines, Gallagher et al. (1994) explored three caregiver characteristics in relation to role overload: the sense of coherence, the manner of coping, and the sense of meaning in the caregiver role. They found that both the sense of coherence (that is, confidence that things would work out) and a feeling of meaning in the caregiver role were related to a positive outcome. On the other hand, the use of situational coping strategies such as being controlling or directive, letting things slide, or using drugs or alcohol was significantly associated with role overload. Novack and colleagues (1991) also found that coping style was related to outcomes.

To summarize from the perspective of the caregiver:

- Caregivers are typically women and are usually the parents or spouse of the disabled care recipient.
- Caregiving is associated with high levels of psychological strain, as well as social, physical, and economic consequences.
- Caregiver strain is related to characteristics of the care recipient, such as the degree and type of disability, and to caregiver characteristics, such as coping style, meaning, and coherence.

Summary

This chapter has presented an overview of the complex topic of caregiving from the perspective of both the caregiver and the care recipient. For professionals working with people aging with disabilities, the messages are clear:

1. Be aware of potential changes in the need for assistance in activities of daily living as clients get older and of the impact of those changes for the individual's sense of independence and quality of life.
2. Remember that receiving assistance makes the client part of a caregiving equation that needs to be balanced on both sides.
3. Enumerate the contributions that clients make to their relationship with the primary caregiver, as a step in maintaining or redressing the balance in that very important relationship.
4. Be aware of the potential for caregiver strain, particularly among caregivers with preexisting psychological problems.
5. Faria (1989) recommended a threefold strategy for supporting caregivers to sustain their participation in the role:

- acknowledge the feelings associated with caregiving;
- find a way of getting the actual caregiving tasks done, which may include enlisting help from others;
- look ahead and have a plan for the future, anticipating the likelihood that the burden of care may increase.

REFERENCES

Arnold, M., and Case, T. 1993. Supporting providers of in-home care: The needs of families with relatives who are disabled. *Journal of Rehabilitation* 59 (1): 55–59.

Bethoux, F., Calmels, P., Gautheron, V., and Minaire, P. 1996. Quality of life of the spouses of stroke patients: A preliminary study. *International Journal of Rehabilitation Research* 19 (4): 291–99.

Bryant, C. S. C. 1993. Understanding decision-making in the caregiving experience of mothers and daughters. Ph.D. diss., University of Virginia.

Coleman, P. D. R. 1993. Determinants of supply of informal care to the frail elderly. Ph.D. diss., Syracuse University.

Faria, S. K. A. 1989. Keep on going: Caregiving by spouses of CVA patients in the home. Ph.D. diss., University of Alabama, Department of Nursing.

Gallagher, T. J., Wagenfeld, M. O., Baro, F., and Haepers, K. 1994. Sense of coherence, coping and caregiver role overload. *Social Science and Medicine* 39 (12): 1615–22.

Gaynor, S .E. 1990. The long haul: The effects of home care on caregivers. *Image—the Journal of Nursing Science* 22 (4): 208–12.

Gerhart, K., Weitzenkamp, D., and Charlifue, S. 1996. The old get older: Changes over three years in aging SCI survivors. *New Mobility* 7 (33): 18–21.

Gillen, R., Tennen, H., Affleck, G., and Steinpreis, R. 1998. Distress, depressive symptoms and depressive disorder among caregivers of patients with brain injury. *Journal of Head Trauma Rehabilitation* 13 (3): 31–43.

Holicky, R. 1996. Caring for the caregivers: The hidden victims of illness and disability. *Rehabilitation Nursing* 21 (5): 247–52.

Holicky, R., and Charlifue, S. 1999. Aging and spinal cord injury: The impact of spousal support. *Disability and Rehabilitation* 21:250–57.

Howe, A. L., Schofield, H., and Hermann, H. 1997. Caregiving: A common or uncommon experience? *Social Science and Medicine* 45 (7): 1017–29.

Kennedy, J., Walls, C., and Owens-Nicholson, D. 1999. A national profile of primary and secondary household caregivers: Estimates from the 1992 and 1993 surveys of income and program participation. *Home Health Care Services Quarterly* 17 (4): 39–58.

Krause, J. S. 1992. Longitudinal changes in adjustment after spinal cord injury: A 15-year study. *Archives of Physical Medicine and Rehabilitation* 73:558–63.

Krause, J. S., and Crewe N. M. 1990. Concurrent and long-term and long-term prediction of self-reported problems following spinal cord injury. *Paraplegia* 28:186–202.

Kulkarni, J. R., Chamberlain, M. A., and Porritt, R. 1992. Dependency in rehabilitation: A comparative study of dependency in hospital and at home. *International Journal of Rehabilitation Research* 15:63–89.

Liu, H. 1991. Factors related to quality of life of Chinese caregivers. Ph.D. diss., University of Illinois at Chicago.

McColl, M. A. 1996. Social support, disability and rehabilitation: A review. *Critical Reviews in Physical and Rehabilitation Medicine* 7 (4): 315–33.

McColl, M. A., Arnold, C., Charlifue, S., and Gerhart, K. 2001. Social support and aging with a spinal cord injury: Canadian and British experiences. *Topics in Spinal Cord Injury Rehabilitation* 6 (3): 83–101.

McColl, M. A., and Skinner, H. A. 1992. Measuring psychological outcomes following rehabilitation. *Canadian Journal of Public Health* 83 (2):s12–s18.

Medeiros, M., Ferraz, M. B., and Quaresma, M. R. 2000. The effect of rheumatoid arthritis on the quality of life in primary caregivers. *Journal of Rheumatology* 27 (1): 76–83.

Mumma, C. M. 2000. Perceived losses following stroke. *Rehabilitation Nursing* 25 (5): 192–95.

Neugarten, B. I., Havinghurst, R. J., and Tobin, S. S. 1961. The measurement of life satisfaction. *Journal of Gerontology* 16:134–43.

Novack, T. A., Bergquist, T. F., Bennett, G., and Gouvier, W. D. 1991. Primary caregiver distress following severe head injury. *Journal of Head Trauma Rehabilitation* 6 (4): 69–77.

Partridge, C., Johnston, M., and Morris, L. 1996. Disability and health: Perceptions of an older sample. *Physiotherapy Research International* 1:17–29.

Periard, M. E. 1989. Perceptual factors in the caregiver-care receiver relationship: Impact of caregiver strain. Ph.D. diss., Michigan State University.

Radloff, L. 1977. The CES-D scale: A self-report depression scale for research in the general population. *Applied Psychological Measurement* 1:385–401.

Schofield, H. L., Hermann, H. E., Bloch, S., Howe, A., and Singh, B. 1997. A profile of Australian family caregivers: Diversity of roles and circumstances. *Australian and New Zealand Journal of Public Health* 21 (1): 59–66.

Schultz, C. L., Smyrnios, K. X., Carrafa, G. P., and Schultz, N. C. 1994. Predictors of anxiety in family caregivers. *Australian Occupational Therapy Journal* 41 (4): 163–61.

Schwartz, L., and Kraft, G. H. 1999. The role of spouse responses to disability and family environment in multiple sclerosis. *American Journal of Physical Medicine and Rehabilitation* 78 (6): 525–32.

Semlyen, J. K., Summers, S. J., and Barnes, M. P. 1998. Aspects of caregiver distress after severe head injury. *Journal of Neurologic Rehabilitation* 12 (2): 53–59.

Stone, R. I., Cafferata, G. L., and Sangl, J. 1987. Caregivers of the frail elderly: A national profile. *Gerontologist* 5:616–26.

Verbrugge, L. M., Rennert, C., and Madans, J. H. 1997. The great efficacy of personal and equipment assistance in reducing disability. *American Journal of Public Health* 87:384–92.

Whiteneck, G. G., Charlifue, S. W., Frankel, H. L., Fraser, M. H., Gardner, B. P., Gerhart, K. A., Krishman, K. R., Menter, R. R., Nuseibeh, I., Short, D. J, and Silver, J. R. 1992. Mortality, morbidity and psychosocial outcomes of persons spinal cord injured more than 20 years ago. *Paraplegia* 30:617–30.

Williamson, J. D., and Fried, L. P. 1996. Characterisation of older adults who attribute functional decrements to old age. *Journal of the American Geriatrics Society* 44:1429–34.

Part 3
Treatment Considerations

6

Maintaining Health and Function

Laura Mosqueda, M.D.

The absence of disease is not the same as good health. Good health implies the presence of positive biological, psychological, social, and spiritual factors. These factors interact to produce an individual's state of health, whether it is good, bad, or somewhere in between. While this chapter will focus on the biological factors involved in maintaining health and function, one must remember that this is only one part of the equation that adds up to good health.

This chapter will discuss how to help a person with a disability maintain health and function. Techniques and interventions for doing so are widely available yet underused by those who are aging with disabilities. As noted in *Healthy People 2010:* "Underemphasis on health promotion and disease prevention activities targeting people with disabilities has increased the occurrence of secondary conditions . . . that a person with a primary disabling condition likely experiences. . . . The health promotion and disease prevention needs of people with disabilities are not nullified because they are born with an impairing condition or have experienced a disease or injury that has long-term consequences" (Centers for Disease Control and Prevention 1999). As people with disabilities age into middle and late life, preventive services and healthy lifestyles become more and more important.

Prevention: Primary, Secondary, Tertiary

Preventing new disease and disability is an important aspect of primary care. There are several types of prevention—primary, secondary, and tertiary— each with special relevance for people with disabilities. Entirely averting a disease through prevention efforts is called primary prevention. The pneumovax, an immunization that keeps an individual from developing pneumococcal pneumonia, is an example of primary prevention: it prevents a disease from occurring. Counseling about the dangers of tobacco use so that a person decides not to start smoking is another example of primary prevention. Both of these interventions (immunizations and counseling) preclude the disease from occurring in the first place. Primary prevention for a person with a disability is especially important. Someone with kyphoscoliosis secondary to cerebral palsy has a decreased lung capacity and so is at risk not only of getting pneumonia, but of having a more difficult time recovering if she does. She ought not wait until she is sixty-five years old to have a pneumovax and yearly flu shot. Instead, she should receive the pneumovax while a young adult, or even during childhood, depending on her risk factors, and should have been receiving a yearly flu shot since young adulthood.

Some diseases may be caught at an early, presymptomatic stage; this is secondary prevention. Treating diseases appropriately at this stage may avoid the accompanying morbidity and mortality that usually occurs without treatment. The use of mammography for a woman who has no evidence of breast cancer (no symptoms, no palpable mass) is an example of secondary prevention. The goal of screening mammography is to find breast cancer at the earliest stage possible so curative therapy can be instituted. Screening colonoscopy is another example of secondary prevention: a person who has no symptoms of colon cancer undergoes a test to look for early evidence of disease. Again, the goal is to provide treatment before the cancer has developed and spread through the lymphatic system.

Some types of secondary prevention, such as the Papanicolaou test (Pap smear) and mammograms, are less likely to be performed if a person has a disability. In an analysis of data derived from the National Health Interview Survey, Iezzoni and colleagues (2001) found that women with moderate or major mobility problems were significantly less likely to have received a Pap smear or mammogram within the past two years than their nondisabled counterparts.

When a person already has a symptomatic disease, there may be ways to prevent or delay associated morbidity and mortality. This is tertiary prevention. People with congestive heart failure, for example, will benefit in two ways from an angiotensin-converting enzyme inhibitor (also called ACE inhibitor): it will reduce symptoms of heart failure and prolong survival. Other forms of tertiary prevention are especially applicable for people who are aging with disabilities. For example, a person with a spinal cord injury who has early osteoarthritis of his shoulders may benefit from lifestyle modifications that will reduce the wear and tear on the joints as well as exercises that will strengthen the musculature and protect the joints. These lifestyle modifications and exercises are a form of tertiary prevention that may allow him many more years of a pain-free and independent life.

Primary Care

A fifty-two-year-old woman with cerebral palsy and mental retardation is severely disabled, both physically and cognitively. She lives with her eighty-four-year-old mother, who continues to be her primary caregiver, as she has been for the past fifty-two years. One day the mother reports that her daughter is having "seizures." This is surprising, since the patient has no history of seizure activity. When asked to describe the "seizures," the mother describes shaking, flushing of the skin, increased spasticity, and a look of discomfort on her daughter's face. Rather than ordering a new medication to control the "seizures," the primary care doctor orders a blood test to look for evidence of the hormonal changes that accompany menopause. These tests are consistent with a menopausal state, and the patient is started on hormone-replacement therapy, thus curing the "seizures."

Finding adequate primary care is relatively straightforward for children; pediatricians are their primary care doctors, and some also specialize in "childhood diseases" such as cerebral palsy, spina bifida, and Down syndrome. But these are no longer just childhood diseases. Most people now live into advanced adulthood with these impairments. While most nondisabled adults have an array of primary care specialists to choose from (family physicians, internists, gynecologists), these primary care specialists receive no routine or required training in dealing with disability. Although many medical programs are trying to rectify this situation, there is no standardized curriculum that focuses on primary care for people with disabilities. Some people argue that physiatrists ought to be the primary care physicians; but physiatrists, who are expert in the area of disability, have almost no required training in primary care. This leaves adults with disabilities in a quandary: whom do they turn to for primary care? While many of the primary care issues are the same for able-bodied people as they are for people with disabilities, some are not. And while many primary care physicians are intimately familiar with the proper primary and preventive care issues for adults, many are intimidated by a patient with a disability. Rather than focusing on the person who needs preventive care, they focus on the disability and miss the person. Thus the basic, yet important, primary care tools that help prevent major illnesses such as cardiovascular disease, cancer, and infections are not provided to people who have disabilities. In one study that reviewed mortality data on people with cerebral palsy, the authors found excess mortality from cancer, stroke, and ischemic heart disease; they postulated that their findings may result from poor surveillance and a lack of early detection (Strauss, Cable, and Shavelle 1999).

Adding strength to the hypothesis that people with disabilities receive poorer primary care than nondisabled people is a study of 101 adults with cerebral palsy (Murphy, Molnar, and Lankasky 1995). All the participants were living in northern California, in the community. More than 90 percent did not have periodic general health evaluations: most of the women had not received regular breast or pelvic examinations; very few of the men had had a prostate examination; and less than 10 percent of the people in the sample had been evaluated for cardiovascular risk factors (hypertension, lipid levels, and fasting blood sugar) (table 6.1). Even when women in this study asked for breast and pelvic examinations, they encountered barriers. The authors explained: "Because of difficulties with inadequate examination room set-up, equipment and with physical limitations resulting from the neuromuscular dysfunction, the examination was often stopped with the mutual consent of the patient and physician."

For adults with mental retardation or brain injuries, cooperating with routine primary care screening may be difficult. Screening for dental, hearing, and visual problems is also important. A person who is losing weight may go through an unnecessary decline and subsequent workup for weight loss simply because no one thought to look for conditions such as dental caries or gingivitis that cause pain with chewing. A person with Down syndrome may have increasing difficulty following directions and then be labeled with Alzheimer disease when in fact he has a severe hearing impairment that was never evaluated. Allied health professionals who are aware of these possibilities play an important role in patient and family education and advocacy. They can encourage people with disabilities to seek care and educate physicians about the

Table 6.1. Primary care for 101 adults with cerebral palsy in the community (mean age = 42.6 years)

No periodic general health examination	90%
No regular breast examination	90%
No regular pelvic examination	90% of women (n = 48)
No digital prostate examination	90% of men (n = 53)
Not screened for CV risk factors (HTN, lipids, glucose)	90%

Source: Adapted from Murphy, Molnar, and Lankasky 1995.

necessity of searching for new, treatable conditions when a decline in function occurs.

Many primary care physicians are not prepared to deal with the multiple and interacting medical, psychological, and social issues that are frequently presented by people who are aging with disabilities. When patients from other populations encounter new or complex problems, they are frequently referred to a comprehensive assessment program. Many such geriatric programs throughout the United States serve older adults. They typically are staffed by an interdisciplinary group of health care professionals, including a primary care physician, physical therapist, social worker, pharmacist, psychologist, nutritionist, and others. The team composition varies owing to practical considerations such as reimbursement and availability of professionals at different institutions. However, there are practically no such programs for people with disabilities, even though their problems are just as complex. One pilot study in England used a comprehensive assessment program to evaluate thirty-eight people with intellectual disabilities. It found that many were overdue for standard health maintenance examinations or procedures and that many had new medical problems that required treatment (Lennox et al. 2001). This particular program also served an important role in educating the primary care providers.

It appears that some barriers to providing high-quality primary care are attitudinal and could be overcome with proper education. Primary care providers must start to think about long-term planning and how to help people with disabilities live long, healthy lives. This means thinking about and discussing preventive health care at all ages, but there are some special issues that arise for people who are aging with disabilities. For example, we may need to think about screening for low bone density when a person with limited mobility is thirty-five years old instead of waiting until she is sixty-five. Since our maximum bone density is achieved by about age thirty and is partially determined by activity level, it stands to reason that a person who has had limited mobility during a time of significant bone formation (childhood and adolescence) may not reach "normal" bone density and thus may be susceptible to fractures as she experiences the gradual bone loss that normally occurs during adulthood. If a thirty-year-old woman with a disability, her physical therapist, and her primary care physician are all thinking about her long-term health, she will be screened for low bone density. Osteopenia or osteoporosis can then be treated at a preclinical stage and save her from experiencing their disabling effects later in life.

Medication Issues

It is not uncommon for people with disabilities to take multiple medications. Often these medications were started when they are young. Some are used to treat the primary impairment, such as the new disease-modifying antirheumatic drugs (DMARDs) and steroids used to treat rheumatoid arthritis. Others are used to treat associated and secondary conditions such as seizures, spasticity, and pain. Still others are used to treat the comorbid conditions such as hypertension and diabetes that are more likely to appear as a person grows older. In many cases patients have been on these medications for years and even decades. We know the danger of long-term use of some medications. For example, chronic use of corticosteroids such as prednisone causes cataracts, obesity, and delayed wound healing. We also know that our ability to eliminate most medications from our body decreases as we age. For example, older adults metabolize and excrete phenytoin (Dilantin) more slowly than younger adults, so a higher concentration of phenytoin circulates throughout the body even though the dosage has remained the same. Even if a person has been on a medication for twenty years with no adverse reactions, it is thus possible for side effects to appear as the person ages because of this change in our ability to metabolize and excrete the drug. In other words, the same dose produces a higher drug level in the body, creating the potential for toxic drug levels (Willcox, Himmelstein, and Woolhandler 1994). It is thus important to understand the basic mechanisms through which medications exert their effects.

To achieve its effects, a drug must be available in adequate concentrations at the appropriate receptors. To achieve this, several steps are involved, including absorption, distribution, biotransformation, and excretion. The best absorption method is the main determinant of how each drug is administered. Oral ingestion is the most common route, but some medications are given by injection, by transdermal patches, or by inhalation. Once in the body, the medication is distributed into the tissues. This distribution is influenced by factors such as the drug's pH gradients, protein binding characteristics, and lipid solubility. Once ingested, a drug undergoes biotransformation, which may render an inactive drug active or vice versa. It may produce metabolites that are also pharmacologically active and may contribute to toxic side effects. Enzymes in the liver are responsible for most biotransformation, but there are also important pathways in the kidneys, lungs, and gastrointestinal tract. Finally, the body must eliminate the drug at approximately the same rate at which it was absorbed in order to achieve the desired effect without toxic effects. The most important organ for eliminating medications is the kidney, although the gastrointestinal system also plays a significant role. These steps of absorption, distribution, biotransformation, and excretion are dependent on factors such as body composition, nutritional status, and comorbid conditions. If any step in this process is altered, the chance of an adverse reaction increases.

People who are aging with disabilities are at particular risk for adverse drug reactions. Physiological differences from their nondisabled counterparts, such as an increase in the fat-to-lean muscle mass ratio in many people with neuromuscular disorders, alters the distribution of some medications in their bodies. Some medications are lipophilic; that is, they preferentially bind to adipose tissue. These medications will have a larger volume of distribution in a person with a disability and will take longer to clear out of the body once they are discontinued. Some people who would benefit from an inhaled medication do not have the dexterity to use an inhaler and are put on oral medications, which generally carry a higher incidence of side effects. People with spinal cord injuries often have concomitant renal disease and may be unable to excrete medications as quickly and efficiently as someone with normal kidney function. So, at the same time that people with disabilities may be on more medications for a longer time, they are also experiencing age-related effects that make them even more susceptible to adverse reactions.

It is thus imperative that all health care providers review the medications that patients are taking (prescription and over-the-counter). A person may be "failing" rehabilitation because of orthostatic hypotension, depression, fatigue, or inability to remember directions. Rather than assuming these problems are secondary to the primary impairment, it is incumbent on members of the health care team to evaluate the medications: all of these signs and symptoms are common side effects of frequently used medications.

> Maria is a sixty-two-year-old woman who has had a complete C-6 spinal cord injury since age twenty-four. She is on multiple medications to treat asthma, pain, depression, glaucoma, and atrial fibrillation. Maria has been on most of these medications for many years and is now having a marked decline in function. Her doctor thinks the decline is an inevitable part of her condition and recommends that she quit her job. Maria requests a therapy evaluation to see if changing her job situation and lifestyle at home might accommodate her changes and improve her function. The therapist sees the long list of medications and recommends a thorough evaluation of her medication regimen. The physician agrees, and it is discovered that three of her medications are no longer needed and one is at toxic levels. When her medication is changed, Maria's function improves dramatically: she is able to think more clearly, is no longer fatigued, and can now take her medications twice a day instead of four times.

Pharmacists are an important and underused resource for evaluating and assessing the dangers of complicated regimens. They also help to simplify dosing schedules, provide patient (and practitioner) education, suggest alternative medications, and analyze risks of medications in individual circumstances.

Transitions

The thought of interacting with a health care provider may be frightening to an adult with a long-term disability.

> A college student with spina bifida did not go to the school's infirmary when he began to feel ill. After a few weeks passed and he continued to get worse, he was too sick to resist going to the doctor. The doctor diagnosed him with pneumococcal (bacterial) pneumonia. This led to a one-week hospital admission for intravenous antibiotics and respiratory therapy followed by four weeks of convalescence at home. His parents asked him why he didn't go to

the doctor sooner; after all, he might have prevented this whole episode had he sought help at the first signs of illness. Eventually, their twenty-two-year-old son told them he was terrified of going to the doctor. The simple act of entering a doctor's office triggered such severe anxiety that he could not even follow through with physical therapy visits because of his dread. The young man described the health care experiences he had when he was growing up with a disability: being poked and prodded by doctors and therapists, and then being poked and prodded again so they could show their students "interesting findings"; having needles stuck in his arm and not understanding why; multiple surgeries that meant separation from his family and friends.

True stories like these help us understand why the thought of interacting with any health care provider may be frightening to an adult with a disability. Fortunately, the care for children with disabilities has changed dramatically, and there is now a much greater emphasis on holistic, family-centered, interdisciplinary care. One hopes that in the future adults will have more positive attitudes about medical care and be better educated about their health care needs.

There are many ways adolescents and young adults can be prepared to make the transition to the adult health care system. The transition may be difficult because holistic, interdisciplinary care is not as available for adults. While there are a few isolated models that provide exemplary care for adults with disabilities, most people are faced with a large, impersonal, and daunting health care system. Therapists and other health care professionals can help patients take an active part in their own health care. We ought to provide explanations, education, and a comfortable environment in which our patients are encouraged to advocate for themselves.

An excellent resource (for both health care professionals and consumers) regarding the transition from child to adult health care is the Health Care Transition Special Interest Group Web site. This service of the Institute for Child Health Policy, funded by grants from the Maternal and Child Health Bureau and the National Institute of Disability and Rehabilitation Research, provides a forum for discussing the challenges of transitioning from pediatric-based to adult-based care. Questions range from practical everyday matters (dealing with nighttime incontinence while traveling) to advocacy (how we might better prepare teens to become independent) to policy issues (setting

up high-quality programs that are accessible) (http://hctransitions.ichp.edu/
programs services.html).

Exercise

The benefits of exercise are well known: good physical fitness reduces the risk
of chronic diseases such as diabetes and stroke, promotes psychological
well-being, and improves function. Other specific benefits include a reduction in blood pressure, an improvement in the HDL/LDL cholesterol ratio, a
reduction in serum triglycerides, an improvement in aerobic endurance, and
weight reduction. We know that among the elderly (including those with
chronic disease and disability) long-term physical activity postpones further
disability and promotes independent living (Spirduso and Cronin 2001).
However, clinicians may not think about the importance of exercise for people with long-term disabilities. Now that this group is living longer, the role of
exercise in maintaining function and delaying the onset of secondary and
comorbid conditions becomes more important. Depending on the type of impairment, presence of concomitant disease(s), and degree of disability, the appropriate mode, duration, and frequency of exercise will vary among individuals (Durstine et al. 2000).

Lack of physical fitness is especially prevalent among adults with mental retardation (Rimmer, Braddock, and Fujiura 1994). In a Canadian study,
thirty-two middle-aged adults and a control group were evaluated for cardiovascular endurance, muscular strength, muscular endurance, flexibility, and
body composition. These parameters were measured at baseline and then thirteen years later. Not unexpectedly, the people with mental retardation had a
lower level of physical fitness than the control group at baseline. A worrisome
finding, however, was that they had a more rapid decline in physical fitness
over time than those without mental retardation (Graham and Reid 2000).

It is important to set reasonable goals and expectations when establishing
an exercise regimen. The person with the disability must be intimately involved in determining the goals as well as the methods to achieve them, and
both may be influenced by the type of impairment as well as local logistics
(such as access to a swimming pool). A person with rheumatoid arthritis may
have goals for strengthening muscles and preventing contractures. A person
with cystic fibrosis may want a protocol that will help fortify respiratory mus-

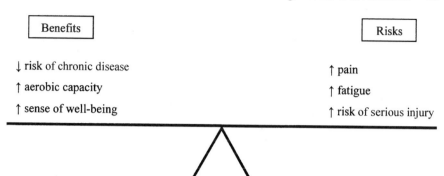

Figure 6.1. Weighing the risks and benefits of exercise: "use it or lose it" versus "conserve it to preserve it."

cles. A person with cerebral palsy may want to focus on increasing range of motion and improving aerobic capacity. A person with mental retardation may view an exercise program as a way to lose weight, increase cardiovascular fitness, and have a new opportunity for socializing.

One concern is that in people with disabilities exercise may do more harm than good. Some people with chromosomal abnormalities (as in Down syndrome) also have atlantoaxial subluxation. This needs to be diagnosed before letting them participate in sports that put stress on the cervical spine, such as diving and soccer. If the pain, fatigue, and weakness that many people experience as they age with disabilities are a function of overuse, then exercise could exacerbate these symptoms. Even though daily activities may put a significant physical strain on the body, this will not improve aerobic capacity unless the effort is sustained for more than fifteen minutes at a minimum of 60 percent of maximum heart rate. Janssen, van Oers, van der Woude, and Hollander (1994) found that middle-aged men with spinal cord injuries, especially those with tetraplegia, experienced episodes of high strain while performing activities of daily living such as transfers and negotiating environmental barriers. However, the only sustained strain occurred during sports. Thus the health care professional needs to help the patient find the level of exercise that will promote cardiovascular conditioning (and other individual goals) yet avoid pain, fatigue, weakness, or injury (fig. 6.1).

An excellent resource for consumers and health care professionals is the National Center on Physical Activity and Disability Web site (www.ncpad.org). The directors of the center provide practical, reliable information about exercise for people with disabilities. Their Web site contains methods of avoiding overuse injuries, cross-training approaches to exercise, fact sheets on exercise for specific impairments, and even information on exercise equipment adapted for people with disabilities.

Falls

Falls are a common and devastating problem as people grow older. There are many reasons for this increase in falls, and it is usually due to a combination of factors rather than to one single factor. Some normal age-related changes such as sarcopenia (loss of muscle mass and strength) and presbyopia (farsightedness) contribute. Medications also frequently contribute to falls; for example, many medications (prescription and over-the-counter) have anticholinergic side effects that result in orthostatic hypotension, blurred vision, and confusion. Many common medical problems such as stroke, diabetes, and macular degeneration increase the risk for falls. Whether it affects the cardiovascular, sensory/nervous, or musculoskeletal system, almost any acute or chronic medical problem can increase a person's risk of falling.

There is limited information in the literature about how common falls are for people who are aging with disabilities. The Rehabilitation Research and Training Center on Aging with a Disability at Rancho Los Amigos National Rehabilitation Center in Downey, California, interviewed 350 adults with disabilities and asked how frequently they fell. Among people with a spinal cord injury or a history of polio, 10–15 percent fell at least once a month, and more than one-third fell at least every two months. The number of falls among people with cerebral palsy was even more alarming: in this group, with an average age of forty-four, 40 percent reported falling at least once a month, and 75 percent fell at least every two months.

As one considers the interaction between normal age-related changes and prior impairment, it is not hard to hypothesize about why the fall rates are so dramatic. Think, for example, about a person with cerebral palsy who struggled to walk as a child. When this person turns forty he now has the accumulated effects of extra wear and tear on his joints (feet, ankles, knees, hips, back) combined with age-related sarcopenia; add in the likelihood of medication-related side effects such as tiring easily and orthostatic hypotension, and it is not surprising that he is a member of the "frequent faller" club.

What is surprising, however, is my own anecdotal experience that people with disabilities do not spontaneously discuss their falls with their health care providers. The reasons are unclear; perhaps the falls have just become an accepted way of life and the person thinks nothing can be done abut them. Whatever the reason(s), it is imperative that health care providers ask about falls, including the frequency and consequences (physical and emotional). If falls are an issue, it is time to do a careful assessment of physical function, assistive devices, home environment, and medications. This is particularly important because the risk of injury from a fall increases with age.

Abuse

People with disabilities have a four to ten times greater chance of being a victim of a crime than people without. Too often this crime involves abuse by a family member, friend, or acquaintance. Although the laws and reporting mechanisms are different from state to state, almost every state mandates that health care providers report abuse to authorities (police, adult protective services, ombudsperson).

The abuse can take any form, from physical abuse by the victim's father to sexual abuse by the school bus driver to financial abuse by a friend to neglect by the in-home caregiver. Manifestations of abuse also take many forms. Bruises, pressure sores, fractures, or poor hygiene may be physical evidence of abuse or neglect. Behavioral changes such as becoming withdrawn, depressed, or agitated may indicate abuse as well.

Physical therapists, occupational therapists, speech and language pathologists, and others on the rehabilitation team spend significant time with their clients and discuss intimate matters. This puts them in an excellent position to notice physical or psychological changes in a client. But these changes may be subtle or easily explained away ("How did I get that bruise? Oh, I just fell") and therefore missed. Many clients, particularly those with mental retardation, may not be able to report or even understand the abusive situation and thus require advocates within the health care system. Health care providers must remain alert that a physical or psychological change may be evidence of abuse and must be willing to ask questions and make a report.

Be aware of the reporting laws in your state. Understand that it is not your duty to investigate, corroborate, or invalidate a suspicion of abuse; it is your duty to make a report if you simply have a reasonable suspicion.

Summary

Now that people with early-onset disabilities are living into middle age and beyond, health promotion and disease prevention are increasingly important. Efforts at primary, secondary, and tertiary prevention will help our patients live long and healthy lives. All members of the health care team must understand the impact of medications and their side effects on clients' health and function. Exercise, one of the most important elixirs for a healthy life, requires a different approach for people who are aging with disabilities and therapists play a key role in assisting with regimens that are safe and effective. Through partnership and coordinated efforts between health care providers and our patients, the possibility of a long, healthy life becomes a reality.

REFERENCES

Centers for Disease Control and Prevention; National Institute on Disability and Rehabilitation Research. 1999. *Healthy People 2010—Conference Edition*, U.S. Department of Education, November.

Durstine, J. L., Painter, P., Franklin, B. A., Morgan, D., Pitetti, K. H., and Roberts, S. O. 2000. Physical activity for the chronically ill and disabled. *Sports Medicine* 30:207–19.

Graham, R., and Reid, G. 2000. Physical fitness of adults with a intellectual disability: A 13-year follow-up study. *Research Quarterly for Exercise and Sports* 71 (2): 152–61.

Iezzoni, L. I., McCarthy, E. P., Davis, R. B., Harris-David, L., and O'Day, B. 2001. Use of screening and preventive services among women with disabilities. *American Journal of Medicine Quality* 16:135–44.

Janssen, T. W., van Oers, C. A., van der Woude, L. H., and Hollander, A. P. 1994. Physical strain in daily life of wheelchair users with spinal cord injuries. *Medicine and Science in Sports and Exercise* 26:661–70.

Lennox, N. G., Green, M., Diggens, J., and Ugoni, A. 2001. Audit and comprehensive health assessment programme in the primary healthcare of adults with intellectual disability: A pilot study. *Journal of Intellectual Disability Research* 45 (3): 226–32.

Murphy, K., Molnar, G. E., and Lankasky, K. 1995. Medical and functional status of adults with cerebral palsy. *Development Medicine and Child Neurology* 37:1075–84.

Rimmer, J. H., Braddock, D., and Fujiura, G. 1994. Cardiovascular risk factor levels in adults with mental retardation. *American Journal Mental Retardation* 98:510–18.

Spirduso, W. W., and Cronin, D. L. 2001. Exercise dose-response effects on quality of life and independent living in older adults. *Medicine and Science in Sports and Exercise* 33:S598–s608.

Strauss, D., Cable, W., and Shavelle, R. 1999. Causes of excess mortality in cerebral palsy. *Developmental Medicine and Child Neurology* 41:580–85.

Willcox, S. M., Himmelstein, D. U., and Woolhandler, S. 1994. Inappropriate drug prescribing for the community-dwelling elderly. *Journal of the American Medical Association* 272: 292–96.

7

Functional Changes Affecting People Aging with Disabilities

Lilli Thompson, P.T.

Most people have a strong desire to maintain optimal function and independence into late life. Preserving health and function throughout the life span has also become a critical concern for people with disabling impairments, because most of them will now live into old age. During the past fifty years, the life expectancy of people with early life impairments has increased faster than that of the general population. However, there is evidence that people with disabilities have reason to be apprehensive about their ability to maintain their hard-won independence. Many are experiencing new functional declines in middle age that threaten this independence, which has become a major issue in the disability community (Corbet 1999). These concerns lead to the following questions: What causes these changes in function? Are there ways to prevent the losses? How can we preserve function as people with disabling impairments age?

This chapter provides an overview of the functional changes that occur in people aging with disabilities and describes some of the factors contributing to these changes. I also discuss ways of assessing functional status, the causes of functional decline, and appropriate interventions and explore the changing needs for assistive technology, personal care assistance, and specific health care services. The new findings suggest additional responsibilities for therapists, including focusing on early detection of symptoms associated with functional loss, providing effective interventions to address functional decline, and implementing strategies to prevent such declines from developing in people aging with disabilities.

The Definition of Function

The term "function" covers a vast spectrum of activities or abilities that are required to accomplish a task or to fulfill a role. The ability to move, to perform basic self-care, to interact with the community, and to maintain social roles are all functional activities. Each of them has many components. For example, mobility includes the ability to move one's body under different conditions or in different environments. Mobility might include the ability to transfer, walk, propel a wheelchair, or drive. activities of daily living (ADLs) include feeding oneself, dressing, toileting, bathing, and grooming. Performing ADLs independently requires the capacity to move and manipulate objects. Instrumental activities of daily living (IADLs) are more complex tasks necessary to live independently in the community. They include shopping, preparing meals, managing medication, doing household chores, and managing finances. Finally, at the far end of the spectrum of function are the broader life roles that include participating in social, recreational, or community activities, parenting, and working. Participating in the life roles usually brings a sense of purpose and meaning to individuals' lives (Kemp 1999). Even so, for individuals each level of function has its own meaning and significance. Therefore clinicians have a responsibility to explore and address functional activities along the spectrum, with special emphasis on the areas that are most important or meaningful to the clients they serve.

Assessing function in a reliable and accurate way is challenging. Clinicians and researchers have used both self-report and performance-based approaches to determine an individual's functional status (Simonsick et al. 2001). Self-report or proxy methods can be inaccurate, and unless sufficient time is devoted to the details of the task performance, clinicians may not acquire critical information. For example, the ability to repeatedly perform a task, difficulty in performing it, changes in performance over time, energy cost, and the customary techniques used to accomplish the task are often not determined from simple self-report questions. Clients also may under- or overestimate function when using self-report means. But self-report or proxy reports may be the only option, and most individuals can provide details of their functional abilities when asked. Performance-based measures have several advantages but at times are impractical. Direct observation of performance in the patients' own environment is ideal but can pose logistical problems for clinicians and researchers. Observation of performance generally requires more time and may require specific environmental setup and equipment if the task is simulated in a clinical setting. Another consideration is the impact that observing performance can have on motivation and effort. The energy or effort required for a task may exceed the individual's daily capacity, but in the testing situation it may be performed anyway. Despite these many considerations, it is still important to obtain an accurate understanding of an individual's functional status. This information is critical to benchmarking changes, directing interventions, and targeting outcomes.

Functional abilities are influenced by the simultaneous interaction of a variety of physical, psychological, and social variables. A person's health status, physical capabilities, organ system capacities, motivation, mental health status, and personal expectations can also influence function, as can the availability of resources and support in the home and community. Living arrangements and the environment or context for performance can also affect function, and with aging the interdependence of these variables increases. Exploring each of these factors and their interrelationships is important when determining a person's functional status and the potential causes of change as one ages. The following sections address physical symptoms that have a negative effect on function and discuss the social and psychological variables that influence functional status (fig. 7.1).

The Effects of Aging on Function

Age-related changes occur in all organ systems throughout one's lifetime. Many of these changes have a direct impact on function, whether or not a person has a preexisting disability. In the nondisabled population, diminished neuromuscular and skeletal integrity can directly affect performance. Sarcopenia (loss of muscle mass and strength), decreased nerve conduction velocity, diminished reflex responses, and changes in sensation all contribute to declines in neuromuscular function in older people (Baumgartner 2000; Hughes et al. 2001). Even a slight decline in force production capacity, delay in response, or loss of sensation can have a significant effect on function in an individual with preexisting movement impairment. In almost any population,

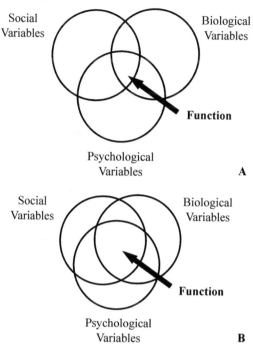

Figure 7.1. A. Function is influenced by the interaction of biological, psychological, and social variables. Kane, Ouslander, and Abrass (1999) described this concept in relation to the
components of a geriatric assessment. The potential interaction of these variables increases
with age and in individuals with a disabling impairment. B. As each variable exerts a greater
influence, a minor change in one factor can have a more significant effect on function.

delays in vestibular response may impair balance and increase the risk of falls.
Decreased elasticity in ligaments and articular surface degeneration can result
in decreased joint flexibility, dysfunction, and pain. Loss of bone mineral density with aging increases the risk of fractures. Age-associated cardiopulmonary
changes including decreased maximal cardiac output, decreased maximal
heart rate, and decreased maximal oxygen consumption can all reduce tolerance for activity. Lung function diminishes with age, as does maximum oxygen uptake (Kane, Ouslander, and Abrass 1999). Each of these organ system
changes has the potential to cause even greater functional decline in people
aging with disabilities.

Despite these age-associated organ system changes, most nondisabled people over age sixty-five perceive their health to be good or excellent (National
Health and Nutrition Examination Survey III 1994; Kane, Ouslander, and

Abrass 1999). Studies confirm that relatively low levels of disability are found in older adults until they reach their mid-seventies. After this, disability rates increase with advancing age and are closely associated with declines in health status. Physical impairments increase and cause functional limitations that create disabilities. For example, a normal and progressive slowing of walking speed has been observed in healthy adults after age seventy (Perry 1992). However, decline in performance is even more pronounced when people with arthritis and other age-related disabilities are included in the analysis. The decline of function may evolve into an actual disability when individuals cannot perform safely or effectively in the community. Another way to identify the onset of changes in functional ability is to note when new needs for assistance with ADLs or IADLs arise. Kennedy, LaPlante, and Kaye (1997) reported that the proportion of the general population who required help with one or more ADLs was 4 percent in the age range sixty-five to seventy-four and 23 percent in people over eighty-five. Disability serious enough to affect ADLs appears to be less common than that affecting IADLs, even in older populations. Kane, Ouslander, and Abrass (1999) reported that in community-dwelling adults over age eighty-five, 40 percent needed assistance with ADLs, while 55-60 percent needed assistance with IADLs. The difference between the two categories likely reflects the different physical or cognitive demands of the tasks. IADLs entail interacting with the community in varied environmental conditions, whereas ADLs can be accomplished in a fairly controlled setting. Another factor to consider is willingness to accept help or the availability of more assistance with IADL tasks rather than the more personal ADL tasks. A general interpretation of the later life declines in function is that organ systems have to deteriorate to relatively low levels before it affects daily function enough to cause disability. These changes eventually affect the ability to live in the community. Estimates are that as low as 7 percent of the population between seventy-five and eighty-four years old lives in long-term care facilities, but this estimate increases to 20 percent in people eighty-five and older (National Hospital Discharge Survey 1996; Kane, Ouslander, and Abrass 1999). The rate of nursing home admissions increases as age advances, primarily because of loss of functional independence, declines in health, and lack of adequate social support.

Functional independence may be threatened at a much earlier age in those with impairments such as cerebral palsy, spinal cord injury, or rheumatoid arthritis. These people already have diminished functioning in key organ systems such as musculoskeletal, neurological, and cardiopulmonary. For some individuals, depending on the age of onset of the disability, organ system capacity may not have ever fully developed during childhood, adolescence, or early adulthood. They thus have a smaller reserve capacity to accommodate to age-associated changes. In addition, a primary impairment may increase susceptibility to secondary health conditions that have additional negative consequences for performance. The combined effect of these factors may substantially reduce an individual's ability to accommodate to the additional "normal" changes associated with advancing age. Even a small decline in physical capacity or health status may have a dramatic effect on the functional status of a person with a disability.

The following sections provide some examples of the interaction of the primary impairment with potential age-associated risks in three specific impairment groups.

Polio

In people with a history of poliomyelitis, residual muscle weakness or frank paralysis may persist throughout the lifetime after the initial acute phase of the disease. Although severe muscle weakness may exist, people with polio generally have intact sensory systems, including proprioceptive and kinesthetic senses. The preserved sensory input has allowed many individuals with polio to function far beyond expectations that are based only on the strength of the muscles in conditions with a lack of proprioceptive sensation. Biomechanically stabilizing joints and using substitution techniques to compensate for weak muscles can enhance functional abilities. Consequently limbs may have been used in ways that exceed their muscle capacity, placing abnormal stresses on joints and weakened muscles. The risk of developing joint pain or joint laxity and of "overusing" muscles increases. The onset of postpolio syndrome, with symptoms of muscle weakness, fatigue, and pain, can mark a rapid and dramatic loss of function that far exceeds normally anticipated aging changes.

Spinal Cord Injury

A spinal cord injury (SCI) disrupts the ascending and descending neural pathways from the brain to the peripheral nervous system, resulting in paralysis and sensory loss below the level of the lesion. A thoracic-, lumbar-, or sacral-level lesion typically causes paraplegia or lower extremity paresis and sensory loss. A cervical-level lesion results in tetraplegia (formerly known as quadriplegia), with paralysis of some of all of the muscles of the arms, hands, trunk, and lower extremities. The degree of cord damage at any given level determines the completeness of the motor and sensory loss below that level. Disruption of the inhibitory input from the central nervous system to the periphery may cause a heightened response of the stretch reflex in the musculotendon complex presenting as muscle spasticity, clonus, or both. Disruption of ascending central pathways from the periphery to the central nervous system affects the assimilation of sensory information. Therefore pain, light touch, temperature appreciation, and kinesthesia may be absent below the lesion. People with SCI are susceptible to multiple health and physical conditions because of the neurological dysfunction.

The combination of the SCI and aging can increase health risks in people with long-term SCI. Loss of sensory input (especially nociceptive afferent stimuli) creates a risk for decubitus ulcers. As skin becomes more fragile with advancing age, this risk increases. Normal voiding is often disrupted by an SCI, resulting in the need for alternative means of managing bowel and bladder function (Young et al. 1996). The gastrointestinal complications, urinary tract infections, and kidney dysfunction associated with SCI are amplified when combined with the age-associated declines in physiological function of these organ systems. Accelerated loss of bone mineral density occurs immediately after SCI and continues throughout the life span. Subsequently, fracture risk increases in osteoporotic bones as people age with SCI (Garland et al. 2001). The impact of a fracture on a person with mobility limitations can be significant. People immobilized on bed rest may experience pressure sores, pneumonia, blood clots, and diminished endurance, while those attempting to stay active have to manage the constraints of an immobilizing device and potential delays in healing.

In the musculoskeletal system of people with SCI, arm, neck, and back pain are commonly reported, owing in part to the abnormal demands on the upper body in people with paralysis (Seelen and Vuurman 1991; Sie et al. 1992; Burnham et al. 1993; Corbet 1999). Atypical musculoskeletal demands combined with aging changes in the musculoskeletal system can create significant functional consequences as people with SCI age.

Cerebral Palsy

Cerebral palsy (CP) is a nonprogressive encephalopathy disrupting motor function that is apparent in children before age five. The degree of motor involvement varies dramatically, from very mild abnormalities in the tone of discrete muscle groups to full body involvement with severe spasticity or athetoid movements. The dysfunction of motor control associated with CP creates excessive physical stress, movement compensations, and biomechanical abnormalities resulting in chronic overuse and atypical use of joints and muscles. Musculoskeletal dysfunction and a high prevalence of pain are reported at relatively young ages in people with CP (Murphy, Molnar, and Lankasky 1995). Contractures, scoliosis, and chronic hip dislocations or subluxations are some of the common conditions individuals with CP manage from early childhood. Additional health concerns developing in midlife include increased prevalence and severity of pain, new occurrence of paresthesias (abnormal skin sensations), increased rates of infections, and new problems with incontinence. Health and physical function are affected by the progression of these conditions as people with CP age (Murphy, Molnar, and Lankasky 1995).

Physical Symptoms Related to Functional Changes

Pain, fatigue, and weakness have commonly been reported in people showing functional decline across a wide variety of impairment groups. The underlying etiologies are generally impairment-specific, but the effects are often similar across groups. These symptoms include new muscle and joint pain, new muscle weakness, and generalized fatigue (Gerhart et al. 1993; Murphy, Molnar, and Lankasky 1995; Halstead 1998; Thompson and Yakura 2001). Despite their high prevalence, the onset of these symptoms should not be considered a "normal" progression of aging with a disability. Instead, new pain, fatigue, or weakness should signal a potentially treatable condition that can be alleviated or minimized with focused interventions. No single condition has been found to explain the occurrence of these symptoms in all impairment groups. A combination of health, physical, social, and psychological factors most likely contributes to their development, and each group has certain susceptibilities related to the particular impairment. For example, recent research indicates that people with SCI have disproportionately high rates of cardiovascular disease, pulmonary dysfunction, genitourinary dysfunction, metabolic disorders, and musculoskeletal degeneration compared with nondisabled populations (Bauman et al. 1999; Linn et al. 2000; Bauman and Spungen 2001). Any one of these health conditions could create secondary impairments. Additionally, new fatigue, pain, or weakness may be an early warning of some of these abnormal health conditions. If these symptoms are considered "just a normal part of aging with a disability" and not thoroughly investigated, these conditions could go undetected and untreated.

Gerhart and colleagues (1993) explored the effect of pain, fatigue, and weakness on ADLs, IADLs, and need for additional assistance in people with SCI. Of a sample of 279 individuals with SCI, 22 percent had new needs for physical assistance as they aged. The additional assistance was first needed at an average age of forty-nine years for those with tetraplegia and fifty-four years for those with paraplegia. High rates of fatigue, weakness, medical problems, and pain were reported in people experiencing this decline in functional status. These same symptoms can make it hard to work and to maintain employment (McNeal, Somerville, and Wilson 1999). Activities requiring high energy, or a full body demand such as bathing, transfers, dressing, household chores, shopping, and preparing meals, were frequently affected by these same symptoms in people with long-standing SCI (Thompson and Yakura 2001).

Pain

A high prevalence of muscle and joint pain has been reported in people aging with disabilities (Halstead and Rossi 1985; Gerhart et al. 1993; Murphy, Molnar, and Lankasky 1995). In the SCI population, reports of pain range from 34 to 94 percent (Siddall, Taylor, and Cousins 1997). Sie and colleagues (1992) studied the prevalence of upper-extremity pain in a group of 239 individuals with SCI who averaged thirty-seven years of age and twelve years after the injury. Fifty-five percent of those with tetraplegia had upper-extremity pain, and 46 percent had shoulder pain specifically. Sixty-four percent of the group with paraplegia had upper-extremity pain, with the most common symptoms associated with carpal tunnel syndrome of the wrists followed by shoulder pain. Studies of the postpolio population report pain prevalence as high as 79 percent (Halstead and Rossi 1985), and pain in the CP population ranges from 23 to 79 percent (Murphy, Molnar, and Lankasky 1995;

Andersson and Mattsson 2001). Of the 179 adults with CP reporting pain in the study by Andersson and Mattsson, 18 percent experienced significant pain daily.

Pain can be a warning symptom of disease or tissue damage. A thorough history and clinical exam is essential to identify the etiology of pain and determine if referral to other health care professionals is necessary. This investigation should include a thorough examination of the musculoskeletal and neurologic systems, a determination of the acuteness and level of irritability of the pain, and an assessment of the typical daily demands placed on the musculoskeletal system. People with movement impairments often use altered biomechanics that create atypical demands on muscles and joints. For example, the high prevalence of shoulder and wrist pain in people with SCI is likely due to the unusual demands on the upper extremities required for mobility. In propelling a manual wheelchair, walking with crutches or a walker, transferring, propping, and raising the body to relieve pressure, the shoulders and wrists must function as weight-bearing joints. Individuals who walk with gait deviations are also susceptible to pain and dysfunction in the low back and lower extremity joints, especially the hips and knees.

The onset of new pain may have an additional disabling effect in people with preexisting mobility impairments. A fairly minor musculoskeletal problem can cause a marked decrease in mobility and functional independence. The Rehabilitation Research and Training Center (RRTC) on Aging with a Disability (Downey, California) investigated the effect of pain on function in various impairment groups. Participants reported the amount of additional disability created by pain for various activities. Individuals with rheumatoid arthritis (RA) had the highest prevalence of pain and the greatest disability resulting from pain. Participants with various musculoskeletal disorders, including fibromyalgia, osteogenesis imperfecta, and myotonic dystrophy had the second highest prevalence of pain and pain-induced disability, followed by people with a history of polio. Pain primarily interfered with self-care, home responsibilities, and family activities in people with RA, polio, SCI, and the varied musculoskeletal disorders. Pain had two to four times more effect on the performance of basic functional tasks in the group with disabling impairments than on a nondisabled control group. The nondisabled group identified recreation as the activity most disrupted by pain. In contrast, disruption of self-care and life support activities was reported by people with a preexisting impairment (unpublished data from the RRTC 2001). These findings suggest that pain added to a preexisting impairment increased the disability in some essential functional areas. For impairment groups such as RA and fibromyalgia, where pain is a hallmark of the condition, these findings may be expected. In contrast, the onset of new debilitating pain in people with CP, polio, or SCI may not have been anticipated either by the medical community or by people with the disability.

Managing and treating pain is a complex process. Typical therapy-based treatment includes manual therapy techniques, therapeutic modalities, therapeutic exercise, and, when appropriate, prescribing of assistive or adaptive equipment. Education and functional retraining to modify activities constitute an important component of treatment to avoid continual reinjury. Pain that is severe, not alleviated by rest, or easily aggravated is considered "highly irritable." It is especially important to focus on preserving range of motion and strength, providing pain relief measures, and encouraging active rest when a person is experiencing such pain. When pain is relieved with rest, responds to therapeutic techniques, occurs only with specific movements, postures, or activities, or is rated as low to mid-range for severity, a slow progression to resume activities while guarding against exacerbation is recommended.

Completely eradicating pain may not be possible, especially when a treatable source cannot be identified or if a chronic pain condition exists. Interventions at this point focus on decreasing the severity of pain and its effect on function. Comprehensive pain management programs traditionally rely on a team approach, including pharmacological interventions, activity and lifestyle modifications, and psychological strategies to cope with pain. Pacing is often recommended to lessen stress and modify pain-provoking activities. Pacing requires setting priorities and reducing nonessential tasks to a manageable level that can be performed as close to pain-free as possible (see exhibit 7.1). Maintaining flexibility in the daily schedule allows for opportunities to monitor pain and adjust activities accordingly. Essential activities may have to be modified and nonessential ones postponed or stopped completely. Incorporating rest breaks during the day, assuming nonpainful positions for some time each day, and performing gentle stretching to promote pain-free movements are examples of some routine pain management strategies.

Treating acute inflammatory conditions in the musculoskeletal system of people with mobility impairments can be complicated owing to the demands of daily functioning. If a painful upper extremity is critical for mobility, the person may not be able to adequately rest the limb without severely limiting

---

Exhibit 7.1. Pacing strategies for managing pain and fatigue

Identify: List activities in each category that contribute to pain or fatigue

    ADLs

    IADLs

    Mobility

    Recreation/social

    Work/school tasks

    Other

Prioritize: Have the individual identify the activities that are meaningful, valuable, or pleasurable.

Emphasize: These are the activities to try to preserve in some form.

Problem solve: Identify how to improve efficiency, modify, or obtain assistance for activities that must continue. Identify how to discontinue activities that are not necessary, meaningful, pleasurable, or of value to the individual.

Maintenance: Continually reassess the list and activities. Make appropriate modifications as necessary.

---

function. If acute conditions are not treated appropriately, progression into chronic dysfunction becomes likely. People with disabilities should be vigilant regarding the development of new pain and seek prompt treatment, which improves the chances of successfully eradicating it.

Pain caused by overuse or atypical use of the musculoskeletal system may respond to changing performance techniques and protecting painful structures. Ongoing investigations detailing the timing and magnitude of forces exerted during specific activities (Mulroy et al. 1996; Perry et al. 1996; Newsam et al. 1999), the effect of muscle strength imbalances on performance (Burnham et al. 1993), and the sources of pain in people with specific impairments (Sie et al. 1992; Curtis et al. 1999; Waters and Sie 2001) provide valuable guidance for effective interventions. Modifying wheelchair and walking ergonomics, changing wheeling and transferring biomechanics, and prescribing specific exercises to strengthen and stretch key muscles and joint structures are the types of clinical interventions suggested from these detailed research investigations.

An individual experiencing shoulder pain with transfers from the wheelchair to the car can illustrate how modifying an activity may assist with pain management. The person used a technique adopted many years ago in which one arm was placed on the roof of the car to lever the body from the wheelchair over to the driver's seat. This technique forces the humeral head upward into the subacromial arch, creating an increased risk for damage to the rotator cuff tendons, causing inflammation and shoulder pain. The intensity and duration of shoulder pain progressively increased until it affected overhead reaching, mobility, and other daily activities. Modifying the technique to a depression style transfer (hands placed down on the seat and lifting the body across the space) or introducing the use of a slideboard reduces the susceptibility of the shoulder to this type of impingement. In addition, strengthening the shoulder depressors and rotator cuff muscles to stabilize the humerus will prevent uncontrolled upward translation of the humerus in the glenoid fossa and decrease the chance of impingement with the new method of transfer. Altering the transfer technique to protect the shoulder can eliminate the cause of the pain while preserving the ability to perform the activity either independently or with equipment assistance. The painful condition will be more likely to respond to therapeutic interventions without constant reinjury. Education about alternative techniques or use of different equipment can decrease the risk of injury to muscles and joint structures as aging changes occur and, in cases of existing injury, make therapeutic interventions more effective.

Fatigue

Lack of energy, inability to perform routine activities, and limited capacity to be up and active are a few of the fatigue-associated descriptions reported by people aging with disabilities. While the onset of new fatigue is a significant problem, it is often difficult to address in clinical as well as research settings. The term "fatigue" itself is confusing and can refer to a variety of symptoms. There are several types of fatigue: central, peripheral, and mental. Central fatigue is a generalized lack of energy, feeling exhausted or tired. If this exhaustion is beyond what is considered reasonable or expected based on an individual's activity level, it is considered abnormal. Peripheral fatigue refers to muscle weakness (the decreased ability to generate force) or lack of muscle endurance (an inability to generate repetitive force). Mental fatigue describes the inability to focus, concentrate, or stay alert.

Although central fatigue is a common symptom presented in a variety of

Exhibit 7.2. Conditions that contribute to fatigue
Disrupted sleep
Medication side effects
Inefficient movement
Deconditioning
Pain
Pulmonary dysfunction
Chronic or recurring infection
Systemic disease (hepatitis, AIDS, lupus, etc.)
Excessive energy demands
Depression
Anemia
Cancer
Thyroid disease
Cardiovascular disorders
Abnormal blood glucose (diabetes, hypoglycemia, etc.)

clinical settings, it is not always fully addressed or investigated (Price et al. 1992; Walker, Katon, and Jenelka 1993). Multiple factors may contribute to fatigue, such as underlying medical conditions, poor diet, inadequate rest, stress, and overwork of the body. Chronic fatigue syndrome, major depression, RA, systemic lupus erythematosus, Lyme disease, malignancy, and multiple sclerosis are just a few of the medical conditions that include fatigue as a major diagnostic feature (Schwartz, Jandorf, and Krupp 1993). (See exhibit 7.2.)

The prevalence of fatigue is estimated to be three times as high in people with disabling impairments as in the general population. The Rehabilitation Research and Training Center on Aging with a Disability (2001) has found fatigue rates ranging from 62 percent to 78 percent in people with CP, RA, polio, and SCI. In comparison, the prevalence of fatigue in the general population ranges from 15 to 20 percent (Price et al. 1992; Walker, Katon, and Jenelka 1993).

Two primary factors may contribute to the fatigue experienced by people with disabilities. First, their physical activities require higher physical demands than for those with no disability (Janssen et al. 1994). Excessive fatigue may result from the high level of chronic physical strain required to perform daily activities. For example, Janssen and colleagues (1994) found excessive and prolonged cardiovascular demands in people with tetraplegia when lifting objects, propelling a wheelchair outdoors, ascending ramps and curbs, showering, and performing car transfers compared with the routine physical demands of a nondisabled population. Second, people with disabilities seem more susceptible to abnormal medical conditions than their nondisabled counterparts. The fatigue may be a symptom of an underlying illness, or it may be a side effect of medication used to treat secondary conditions.

Fatigue is an extremely debilitating condition. Reports from people with disabilities who experience fatigue provide a glimpse of the insidious and pervasive cost it exacts from daily function. In the early phases of fatigue, many people say they manage by giving up meaningful activities such as recreation, social outings, or anything considered "extra" in an effort to preserve work, self-care, and IADLs (unpublished data from the RRTC 2001). Eventually fatigue may interfere with these tasks as well. Fatigue has been identified as a reason for early retirement or, for older individuals, decisions to give up work completely (McNeal, Somerville, and Wilson 1999; Krause 2001). As fatigue progresses, it can interfere with home and self-care activities. To conserve declining energy, people with various impairments report limiting the hours they are up and reducing their activities throughout the day. Examples include staying in bed later in the morning or lying down in the afternoon or evening to rest the body, not necessarily to sleep. Some people with postpolio syndrome report that fatigue and lack of energy dictate every aspect of their lives and every decision they make. This becomes so severe that once they determine they have enough energy to attempt an activity, they must next consider what price they will pay to recover afterward.

Ongoing research being conducted by the RRTC on Aging with a Disability is investigating the effect fatigue has on physical function in people with disabilities. A fatigue questionnaire was administered to 206 participants with disabilities who were experiencing central fatigue. Of the 105 participants with polio, 77 percent experienced central fatigue and 59 percent identified fatigue as their most disabling condition, while 83 percent ranked it among the top three. Fatigue takes a toll in people with other impairments as well. Fatigue was reported to prevent sustained physical function in 100 percent of the people with RA, 98 percent of those with CP, 87 percent of those with polio, and 65 percent of those with SCI. Fatigue interfered with duties and responsibilities in the lives of two-thirds of the group with CP and SCI and over one-fourth of the polio group. Participants with disabilities had fatigue severity ratings comparable to ratings reported by Schwartz, Jandorf, and Krupp (1993) for people with chronic fatigue syndrome, multiple sclerosis, systemic lupus erythematosus, and post-Lyme disease.

The general approach to treating fatigue is similar to that described for pain. The underlying cause must first be investigated. New generalized fatigue that is interfering with daily function has to be considered abnormal. Inquiring about changes in energy level and the presence of fatigue as part of routine screenings acknowledges the potential for developing fatigue and provides an opportunity to explore the problem. After an evaluation and diagnosis, the client and health care provider can make informed decisions about the best course of treatment and management. Finding mechanisms to reduce fatigue and minimize its impact on function is an important treatment goal.

Changes in lifestyle are often recommended to conserve energy. When setting priorities, individuals should identify the activities that enhance their overall quality of life and which ones they consider most meaningful and valued. Modifying these valued activities may be necessary, but the primary goal should be to try to preserve them in some form. Individuals are encouraged to save energy for the most meaningful activities by improving the efficiency of supportive activities and by getting help with the daily tasks that demand high energy. For instance, if bathing and dressing are performed more efficiently with assistance (either from equipment or from another person), enough energy may be conserved for participation in personally important community, family, or social activities. Another common example is walking. All too frequently, pleasurable community activities cease because walking has become too fatiguing. However, people may reject a recommended mobility device because a cane, brace, powered wheelchair, or scooter looks too "disabling." The device could decrease the fatigue caused by walking and enhance mobility, thereby actually decreasing the "disability." In hindsight, many people wonder why they resisted accepting new technology once they get used to it.

Minimizing movement dysfunction can enhance efficiency and reduce fatigue. Providing appropriate stability and adequate freedom of movement can decrease energy expenditure. A stable base for movement at the shoulder girdle, trunk, and pelvis and adequate stability in the extremities to meet weight-bearing demands are important components of efficient movement. Muscle weakness, poor physical endurance, and joint laxity contribute to instability in the limbs and trunk. Minimizing spasticity, joint contractures, excess muscle tone, and pain that interfere with free, fluid movement promotes efficiency. In some cases adding custom-designed functional orthoses or postural support devices can provide the stability necessary to reduce pain, optimize posture, or support joints.

Managing fatigue through pacing and lifestyle modification is an ongoing learning process that requires practice and patience. A strategy recommended by Halstead (1998) has a certain appeal. He suggests that instead of giving up entire activities that are meaningful, people try making many small energy conservation changes throughout the day. The accumulation of conserved energy may have a relatively large payoff in reducing fatigue. For example, improving mobility, getting help with chores, and taking periodic rest breaks during the day may conserve more energy than if a major meaningful activity is stopped altogether. If the activities most important to an individual are preserved, the quality of life may be sustained despite significant changes in function.

Weakness

Reports of new muscle weakness are found across multiple impairment groups as people age with a disability (Halstead and Rossi 1985; Gerhart et al. 1993; Murphy, Molnar, and Lankasky 1995; Bursell, Little, and Stiens 1999). Weakness, or the loss of force production capacity of a muscle or muscle group, has been documented in multiple studies of people with postpolio syndrome and rheumatoid arthritis (Grimby et al. 1998; Klein et al. 2000). Subjective measures or self-reports of feeling weaker are documented in studies of aging in people with SCI and CP (Gerhart et al. 1993; Murphy, Molnar, and Lankasky 1995; Thompson 1999). In a sample of 150 people with an average duration of SCI of thirteen years, 11 percent attributed declines in function to a new loss of muscle strength (Thompson and Yakura 2001). New neurologic abnormalities, metabolic dysfunction, or development of a deconditioned state, among other causes, may explain new weakness.

Other contributors to declines in muscle performance include sarcopenia, joint or muscle pain, and deconditioning of muscle groups. With advancing age, a decrease in the muscle mass and the number and size of muscle fibers has been associated with declines in muscle contractile strength. Recent investigations also suggest the need to explore other cellular, neural, and metabolic mediators of strength loss with aging (Hughes et al. 2001). Muscles weakened by deconditioning generally are responsive to the same types of strengthening principles applied to able-bodied populations. However, when determining what types of exercises are appropriate, special consideration is necessary for muscle groups affected by peripheral or nerve root injury or those susceptible to overuse syndromes. This is particularly true in the polio population because of postpolio syndrome.

People often first recognize a loss of strength when they cannot perform a regular functional task. Upper extremity weakness is frequently associated with an inability to lift objects. For individuals with disabilities, arm weakness can affect the ability to lift body weight for transfers, propel a wheelchair, or manipulate objects with their hands. If there is weakness of the lower extremities, they may have difficulty rising from a chair or climbing stairs or inclines, or they may fall frequently. Clinicians should specifically question patients about changes in ability and probe for details, because it is not uncommon for individuals to just accommodate to the changes or minimize their importance. A report of difficulty in performing a once routine task or a report of falls should be a red flag to investigate changes in muscle function.

Age-associated declines in muscle strength and endurance that are super-imposed on preexisting muscle weakness may significantly affect mobility. The strength required for physical performance relates to the force production demand on a muscle or muscle group, the energy cost of the specific activity, and the individual's functional capacity and neuromuscular integrity. Each of these factors must be considered when investigating how new muscle weakness affects function. As an example, consider the effect of isolated pretibial muscle weakness on walking. If the pretibials have only a 3+/5 grade (fair plus) the muscles have the ability to raise the foot upward (dorsiflex) through the full range of motion against gravity and hold against a minimal amount of resistance for at least one single repetition. As the foot touches the ground, the demand on the pretibials is twofold, first to control how fast the foot is lowered to the floor after heel contact and then to move the body weight forward from the heel to the forefoot. In the swing phase the pretibials raise the foot back up to a neutral position to assist with limb clearance. A weakened pretibial muscle group may require a near maximum capacity exertion with every step. It is unlikely this muscle group would have sufficient endurance to meet this demand for very long before gait deviation would occur, affecting limb clearance and forward progression. The deviations and the resulting compensation strategies are energy consuming. Such a force demand that is near or beyond a single muscle group's capacity can rapidly drain existing strength and impair the muscle's ability to perform its necessary role. Instability, increased energy expenditure, and loss of function may result.

New weakness in multiple muscle groups in individuals with preexisting weakness also increases fatigue and causes additional pain and loss of critical function. For example, the combination of calf and quadriceps muscle weakness can have a negative effect on walking. The calf muscles provide an important stabilizing force during stance. If the calf muscles (soleus) are weak, a greater demand is placed on the quadriceps to stabilize the leg. If the quadriceps also becomes weak, the knee may collapse when it is unable to support body weight. To compensate for the instability, individuals might try to biomechanically lock the knee in extension (by keeping body weight ahead of the knee joint), dramatically shorten their step length, slow their walking speed, or use an assistive device for more stability. People whose leg muscles lack enough force production capacity or endurance to meet the highly repetitive demands of walking will display energy consuming gait deviations or experience dire consequences such as a falls. Appropriate leg bracing can often provide the tibial control necessary to restore stance stability and normalize heel off and step length.

The choice to continue walking is affected by pain, fatigue, and movement inefficiency. A study of individuals with CP by Murphy, Molnar, and Lankasky (1995) found that 75 percent of the individuals who stopped walking by age thirty did so because of excess fatigue, inefficient walking, and the improved function they got from a wheelchair. By age fifty, an additional 12 percent had stopped walking because of painful joints and fatigue. Lack of selective muscle control impairs a person's ability to modulate the intensity and timing of a muscle's action. Muscle weakness may underlie the deficits in selective control in people with cerebral palsy, stroke, brain injury, spinal cord injury, and multiple sclerosis. For some, mass pattern movements are useful for gross motor function. New muscle weakness that decreases volitional control can make it hard to initiate a patterned movement or to break through a pattern and use a muscle selectively. On one hand, an increase in spasticity can disrupt control of the timing to initiate or inhibit muscle activity, while a decrease in spasticity may uncover significant underlying volitional muscle weakness. A muscle group may not have sufficient volitional strength to perform a movement that was previously accomplished through the aid of spasticity. Thus, changes in spasticity, whether increased or decreased, among people aging with disabilities can have a significant impact on function.

Bracing to support joints and protect weakened muscles preserves functional use of extremities (Perry 1992; Perry and Clark 1997). In specific cases, appropriately designed lower extremity orthoses provide the stance stability, forward progression, and limb clearance necessary for walking. Wrist-hand orthoses maintain certain hand functions when weakness is present. The variability of hand size and shape and the movement precision required for hand function usually make customized hand orthoses necessary. Custom designed bracing is usually necessary to meet the unique needs of people with disabling impairments. "Off the shelf" orthoses generally do not address the specific requirements for each individual. For example, a generic orthosis to prevent foot drop may fit poorly and create skin ulcers in insensate skin. Furthermore, if this brace is inappropriately used to address calf weakness, it usually is not rigid enough to prevent tibial collapse in stance and therefore is ineffective.

Exercise Considerations

The health benefits from exercise suggest that determining how much is necessary, how to exercise, and even if exercise is appropriate are valid questions for people aging with disabilities. The significant physical and psychological benefits obtained from regular exercise cannot be denied. Cardiopulmonary function, musculoskeletal strength, endurance, overall energy reserves, and mood can be enhanced through safe, effective exercise. How to balance the need for physical activity to promote health against concerns about overtaxing a musculoskeletal system and adding more physical work to individuals already functioning near maximum capacity for daily activities is just one of many underlying questions.

Exercise can help people maintain health, prevent injury, and regain optimal performance. But physical conditioning for cardiovascular and musculoskeletal health, such as muscle stretching, strengthening, and aerobic exercise, should be crafted specifically to match the individual's needs and abilities. The stability of surrounding joints and functional demands of targeted muscle groups must be considered in muscle strengthening regimens. Adding more demands on joints with abnormal biomechanics or muscles functioning at near peak capacity for routine daily functions may be detrimental. Muscle imbalances may be exacerbated if muscle groups are already meeting high force production demands. Working muscles in modes other than those required for daily function decreases the potential for overuse and avoids exacerbating muscle imbalances while achieving the desired health benefits. Performing strengthening exercises using different motions than those required for primary mobility should be encouraged. Curtis and colleagues (1999) identified a relative weakness of the adductors and internal rotators of the shoulder in wheelchair athletes with shoulder pain. Selective strengthening of these muscle groups to restore the balance of muscle strength enhanced shoulder girdle function. Upper extremity or combined upper and lower extremity cycle ergometry can change the orientation and use of the limbs and trunk muscles while promoting cardiopulmonary health. Aquatic exercise with appropriate safety precautions makes use of the buoyancy and resistance of the water with virtually unlimited planes of motion. Postural support muscles can be activated or rested while working specific muscle groups. Depending on the individual's response to water and temperature, tone and spasticity interference can be minimized and pain reduced in weight-bearing joints.

Providing a mode of exercise different from the means used for mobility is important. Functional mobility should maintain the fundamental goal of efficient movement. In contrast, the goal of exercise is to stress a system to increase the reserve capacity for daily function or athletic performance. Most exercise strategies used in the able-bodied population do not rely solely on performance of ADLs and IADLs or general mobility to achieve this goal. Even when members of the general population use walking to keep fit, they make a conscious effort to exercise and use proper equipment (walking shoes). In people with movement impairments, using an inefficient means of mobility for exercise may cause injury, limit their functioning, and ultimately decrease overall physical activity. For example, if walking from the parking lot to the job, the store, or a friend's home becomes a major cardiovascular effort or increases pain, eventually people will stop because of the exceptional strain. Instead, exercise should be performed as a conscious choice using appropriate equipment and with environmental needs met. This philosophy requires health care providers to explore, prescribe, support, and guide individuals with disabilities in their access to programs, equipment, and knowledge about exercise.

New Needs

Age-related changes in health and function create new support needs for people with disabling impairments (Campbell, Sheets, and Strong 1999). Additional functional limitations result in changing equipment needs and new or increased demands for personal care assistance. Dramatic changes in living situations may be required if support needs go unmet. If individuals cannot maintain independence at home and if social supports to meet care needs are inadequate, the ultimate consequence may be some form of assisted living, regardless of age. When technology, home support services, educational opportunities, and environmental access are adequate, individuals with very significant impairments can maintain independent living, achieve productive, competitive employment, and have a high quality of life.

People experiencing declines in function may try to accommodate to changes on their own. Often they will try to adapt themselves to the environment rather than adapting the environment to their new or changing needs. These strategies may work as stopgap measures for a short time. Contact with health care providers usually becomes necessary when self-styled interventions are no longer successful. Health care professionals should take advantage of every opportunity to screen for changes or declines in function. Asking key questions about functional status, the presence of new symptoms, and needs for assistive devices can uncover issues that would benefit from early intervention. Individuals may be unaware of new technology or benefits available to them as they age and change with a disability. Often people underestimate their need for new equipment or do not know they are eligible for services, such as vocational rehabilitation or in-home support, that could maintain their abilities with work, ADLs, and IADLs (McNeal, Somerville, and Wilson 1999).

Equipment needs change throughout the life span of individuals with early life impairments. People aging with disabilities need access to technology to meet these changing needs. Equipment used in childhood or provided during initial rehabilitation may no longer be safe or appropriate. The lack of proper equipment for use by adults with cerebral palsy discovered in a study by Murphy, Molnar, and Lankasky (1995) is alarming. Only two of seventy-eight people with moderate to severe dysarthria (difficulty articulating words) had augmentative communication devices. Ninety percent of the assistive devices for walking were wrong in either fit or function. Only one person out of thirty-four ambulators had a leg orthosis that fit correctly. Only three people out of sixty-seven had any form of postural support on their wheelchairs; the rest had poorly fitted sling seats. These findings create particular concern because of the high prevalence of scoliosis, postural deformity, joint pain, and fatigue in people with CP. Furthermore, even simple wheelchair seating systems for individuals with disabilities can enhance function and reduce musculoskeletal pain. An individual's body size, posture, strength, and the functional requirements for a wheelchair all change with age. Changes in mobility devices, bathing and toileting equipment, computer technology, and home and work accommodations and the addition of ADL assistive devices are just a few examples of new needs that arise as functional capacities change with age. Special considerations apply to mobility equipment, and customized designs may be indicated. For example, maintaining a lightweight, portable wheelchair design is important and has to be considered along with the need for additional postural supports that add weight.

People may be reluctant to accept recommended equipment if they see it as a sign of failure, increased dependence, or increased disability. To counter this perception, new equipment should be presented as technology that decreases disability and enhances function. Recommendations may have to be presented several times before a person is ready to consider using new technology. Ultimately the choice to use or reject the technology should rest with the consumer and not reflect a lack of access to appropriate equipment.

Providing equipment options as soon as the need is anticipated may encourage acceptance of new assistive devices. For example, if a powered wheelchair is indicated in the near future, making the chair available when it is needed only part time might minimize resistance to its use. Similar strategies may be helpful when a person is transitioning from walking to a manual wheelchair or powered scooter. An abrupt shift in the primary means of mobility can be difficult before all the implications have been considered. A few examples of issues to be addressed when equipment changes take place include how to transport a powered wheelchair or scooter; what accommodations are required owing to the height differences between different types of wheelchairs (manual versus powered); and what additional accommodations are necessary for accessibility to various environments when walking, wheeling, or using powered means (e.g., new ramps, handrails, or elevators).

In the aging nondisabled population, the resources available for personal care are an important determinant of the ability to live successfully in the community. Family and close friends provide most of the caregiving both in the general population and for those with disabling impairments. It has been estimated that family members bear approximately 80 percent of the caregiving responsibilities for people aging with disabilities (Seelman 1999). These responsibilities include meeting physical, psychological, emotional, and financial needs. Studies have shown that as function changes with age, the family is called on for help even more frequently in individuals with disabilities (Thompson and Yakura 2001). An increased reliance on family members may become a problem as spouses and parents face their own age-related health and functional changes. When consumers seek paid assistance, they need new skills and knowledge to hire and manage personal care providers.

Summary

Recent investigations have given us a better understanding of the functional loss in people aging with preexisting impairments. Future research will better establish the links to underlying medical conditions. The causes of functional declines are usually complex. Underlying medical illnesses, wear and tear, abnormal psychological factors, social issues, and pharmacological problems can all contribute in varying degrees. As underlying medical conditions and associated factors of pain, fatigue, weakness, and other secondary conditions are determined, early interventions may minimize the impact and slow the rate of functional decline.

From the rehabilitation perspective, understanding the causes and prevalence of later life functional problems is a priority. Rehabilitation clinicians have the unique role of preventing future problems by modifying early rehabilitation practices and by providing early intervention for new problems through a continuum of outpatient services. Rehabilitation philosophies based on preparing individuals for a long, healthy life should incorporate a balance of some of the following: identifying efficient mobility means that optimize and protect musculoskeletal function; promoting exercise for health benefits that is safe for the neuromuscular and musculoskeletal systems; and educating patients and their family members or care providers about prevention and treatment options for functional change.

Medical specialists in nonrehabilitation settings should also understand the changing health and functional issues of individuals aging with disabilities. Middle-aged and older adults with long-term disabilities require a broad range of services from a variety of practitioners. Providers in all medical services, ranging from acute care to outpatient orthopedic specialty care, can contribute to health promotion and disease prevention to maintain function. Health maintenance practices for people with disabilities may vary in scope and timing from those for people who are not disabled. For example, screening for health problems at younger ages, expanding access to rehabilitation specialists, and giving access to technology are often considered exceptions to current managed care services (DeJong and Sutton 1998). To maximize health and function in people with disabilities, the exceptions may need to become the standard of good comprehensive care in at-risk groups.

Important preparation for people aging with disabling impairments include gaining knowledge about pertinent health risks and learning to recognize changes in health and function; developing a partnership with primary and specialty health care providers; obtaining knowledge and skills to acquire personal care assistance and new technology; and developing both personal and financial plans that consider changes in function.

REFERENCES

Andersson, C., and Mattsson, E. 2001. Adults with cerebral palsy: A survey describing problems, needs, and resources, with special emphasis on locomotion. *Developmental Medicine and Child Neurology* 43:76–82.

Bauman, W. A., and Spungen, A. M. 2001. Body composition in aging: Adverse changes in able-bodied persons and in those with spinal cord injury. *Topics in Spinal Cord Injury Rehabilitation* 6 (3): 22–26.

Bauman, W. A., Spungen, A. M., Adkins, R. H., and Kemp, B. J. 1999. Metabolic and endocrine changes in persons aging with spinal cord injury. *Assistive Technology* 11:88–96.

Baumgartner, R. N. 2000. Body composition in healthy aging. *Annals of New York Academy of Science* 904:437–48.

Burnham, R. S., May, L., Nelson, E., Steadward, R., and Reid, D.C. 1993. Shoulder pain in wheelchair athletes: The role of muscle imbalance. *American Journal of Sports Medicine* 21:239–42.

Bursell, J. P., Little, J. W., and Stiens, S. A. 1999. Electrodiagnosis in spinal cord injured persons with new weakness or sensory loss: Central and peripheral etiologies. *Archives of Physical Medicine and Rehabilitation* 80:904–9.

Campbell, M. L., Sheets, D., and Strong, P. S. 1999. Secondary health conditions among middle-aged individuals with chronic physical disabilities: Implications for unmet needs of services. *Assistive Technology* 11:105–22.

Corbet, B. 1999. Aging with a disability: What's it like? *New Mobility* 4:22–33.

Curtis, K. A., Drysdale, G. A., Lanza, D., Kolbar, M., Vitolo, R. S., and West, R. 1999. Shoulder pain in wheelchair users with tetraplegia and paraplegia. *Archives of Physical Medicine and Rehabilitation* 80:453–57.

DeJong, G., and Sutton, J. 1998. Managed care and catastrophic injury: The case of spinal cord injury. *Topics in Spinal Cord Injury Rehabilitation* 3 (4): 1–16.

Garland, D. E., Adkins, R. H., Rah, A., and Stewart, C. A. 2001. Bone loss with aging and the impact of SCI. *Topics in Spinal Cord Injury Rehabilitation* 6 (3): 47–60.

Gerhart, K. A., Bergstrom, E., Charlifue, S. W., Menter, R. R., and Whiteneck, G. G. 1993. Long-term spinal cord injury: Functional changes over time. *Archives of Physical Medicine and Rehabilitation* 74:1030–34.

Grimby, G., Stalsberg, E., Sandberg, A., and Sunnerhagen, K. S. 1998. An 8-year longitudinal study of muscle strength, muscle fiber size, and dynamic electromyogram in individuals with late polio. *Muscle and Nerve* 21:1428–37.

Halstead, L. S. 1998. *Managing post-polio: A guide to living well with post-polio syndrome.* Arlington, Va.: ABI Professional Publications.

Halstead, L. S., and Rossi, C. D. 1985. New problems in old polio patients: Results of a survey of 539 polio survivors. *Orthopedics* 8:845–50.

Hughes, V. A., Frontera, W. R., Wood, M., Evans, W. J., Dallal, G. E., Roubenoff, R., and Fiatarone Singh, M.A. 2001. Longitudinal muscle strength changes in older adults: Influence of muscle mass, physical activity and health. *Journal of Gerontology: Biological Sciences* 56A (5): B209–17.

Janssen, T. W. J., Van Oers, C. A. J. M., Van der Woude, L. H. V., and Hollander, A. P. 1994. Physical strain in daily life of wheelchair users with spinal cord injuries. *Medical and Science in Sports and Exercise* 26:661–70.

Kane, R. L., Ouslander, J. G., and Abrass, I. B. 1999. *Essentials of Clinical Geriatrics,* 4th ed. New York: McGraw-Hill.

Kemp, B. J. 1999. Quality of life while aging with a disability. *Assistive Technology* 11 (2): 158– 63.

Kennedy, J., LaPlante, M. P., and Kaye, H. S. 1997. Need for assistance in the activities of daily living. *Disability Statistics Abstract* 18:1–4.

Klein, M. G., Whyte, J., Keenan, M. A., Esquenazi, A., and Polansky, M. 2000. Changes in strength over time among polio survivors. *Archives of Physical Medicine and Rehabilitation* 81:1059–64.

Krause, J. S. 2001. Aging and self-reported barriers to employment after spinal cord injury. *Topics in Spinal Cord Injury Rehabilitation* 6 (3): 102–15.

Linn, W. S., Adkins, R. H., Gong, H., and Waters, R. L. 2000. Pulmonary function in chronic spinal cord injury: A cross-sectional survey of 222 Southern California adult outpatients. *Archives of Physical Medicine and Rehabilitation* 81 (6): 757–63.

McNeal, D. R., Somerville, N. J., and Wilson, D. J. 1999. Work problems and accommodations reported by persons who are post-polio or have a spinal cord injury. *Assistive Technology* 11:137–57.

Mulroy, S. J., Gronley, J. K., Newsam, C. J., and Perry J. 1996. Electromyographic activity of shoulder muscles during wheelchair propulsion by paraplegic persons. *Archives of Physical Medicine and Rehabilitation* 77:187–93.

Murphy, K. P., Molnar, G. E., and Lankasky, K. 1995. Medical and functional status of adults with cerebral palsy. *Developmental Medicine and Child Neurology* 37:1075–84.

National Health and Nutrition Examination Survey III. 1994. U.S. Department of Health and Human Services Center for Disease Control and Prevention, National Center for Health Statistics.

National Hospital Discharge Survey. 1996. U.S. Department of Health and Human Services Center for Disease Control and Prevention, National Center for Health Statistics.

Newsam, C. J., Rao, S. S., Mulroy, S. J., Gronley, J. K., Bontrager, E. L., and Perry, J. 1999. Three dimensional upper extremity motion during manual wheelchair propulsion in men with different levels of spinal cord injury. *Gait and Posture* 10:223–32.

Perry, J. 1992. *Gait analysis: Normal and pathologic function.* New York: Charles B. Slack.

Perry, J., and Clark, D. 1997. Biomechanical abnormalities of post-polio patients and the implications for orthotic management. *Neurologic Rehabilitation* 8:119–38.

Perry, J., Gronley, J. K., Newsam, C. J., Reyes, M. L., and Mulroy, S. J. 1996. Electromyographic analysis of the shoulder muscles during depression transfers in subjects with low-level paraplegia. *Archives of Physical Medicine and Rehabilitation* 77:350–55.

Price, R. K., North, C. S., Wessely, S., and Fraser, V. J. 1992. Estimating the prevalence of chronic fatigue syndrome and associated symptoms in the community. *Public Health Report* 107:514–22.

Rehabilitation Research and Training Center on Aging with a Disability. 2001. Natural Course Study of Aging with a Disability. Downey, Calif. (unpublished data).

Schwartz, J. E. Jandorf, L., and Krupp, L. B. 1993. The Measurement of fatigue: A new instrument. *Journal of Psychosomatic Research* 17 (7): 753–62.

Seelen, H. A. M., and Vuurman, E. F. P. M. 1991. Compensatory muscle activity for sitting posture during upper extremity task performance in paraplegic patients. *Scandinavian Journal of Rehabilitation Medicine* 23:89–96.

Seelman, K. 1999. Aging with a disability: Views from the National Institute on Disability Rehabilitation Research. *Assistive Technology* 11:84–87.

Siddall, P. J., Taylor, D. A., and Cousins, M. J. 1997. Classification of pain following spinal cord injury. *Spinal Cord* 35:69–75.

Sie, I. H., Waters R. L., Adkins, R. H., and Gellman, H. 1992. Upper extremity pain in the post-rehabilitation spinal cord injured patient. *Archives of Physical Medicine and Rehabilitation* 73:44–48.

Simonsick, E. M., Kasper, J., Guralnik, J. M., Bandeen-Roche, K., Ferrucci, L., Hirsch, R., Leveille, S., Rantanen, T., and Fried, L. P. 2001. Severity of upper and lower extremity functional limitation: Scale development and validation with self-report and performance-based measures of physical function. *Journal of Gerontology: Social Sciences* 56B (1): S10–19.

Thompson, L. 1999. Functional changes in persons aging with spinal cord injury. *Assistive Technology* 11:123–29.

Thompson, L., and Yakura J. 2001. Aging related functional changes in person with spinal cord injury. *Topics in Spinal Cord Injury Rehabilitation* 6 (3): 69–82.

Walker, E. A., Katon, W. J., and Jenelka, R. P. 1993. Psychiatric disorders and medical care utilization among people in the general population who report fatigue. *Journal of General Internal Medicine* 8:436–40.

Waters, R. L., and Sie, I. H. 2001. Upper extremity changes with SCI contrasted to common aging in the musculoskeletal system. *Topics in Spinal Cord Injury Rehabilitation* 6 (3): 63–70.

8

The Therapist's Role
in Maintaining Employment

Susanne M. Bruyère, Ph.D., CRC, William A. Erickson, M.S.,
Dorothy J. Wilson, O.T.R., FAOTA, and Nancy Somerville, B.S.

Work is an important part of the identity and economic well-being of most Americans. Being able to work productively into our later years is increasingly a goal for Americans as we live longer and need income to support these extra years. This goal may be more difficult to achieve for someone aging with a disability. This chapter discusses the particular issues related to employment for individuals aging with disabilities and the implications for rehabilitation professionals who provide services to them. We focus on the two main concerns of people with disabilities: getting employed and staying employed. The first is a long-standing problem, but the second is new, because we have only recently begun to appreciate the extent of midlife changes in the health and function of people who have disabilities. In the introductory section, we present information about the labor force participation rates of people with disabilities and about aging workers with disabilities. In subsequent sections we discuss studies done by Cornell University and Rancho Los Amigos National Rehabilitation Center and their implications for rehabilitation practitioners and therapists.

Labor Force Participation Rates of People with Disabilities

Approximately one in five people has a disability (Stoddard et al. 1998), yet people with disabilities are greatly underemployed or unemployed compared with their nondisabled peers. In the United States in 1999, 34 percent of men and 33 percent of women with disabilities were employed, compared with 95 percent of men and 82 percent of women without disabilities (U.S. Bureau of the Census 2000). This represents a significant loss of willing and able talent to both private- and public-sector organizations, as well as a loss of income and social and economic participation for people with disabilities. This disparity results from inequities in social policy, access to education, training, and employment as well as from society's attitudes.

As the workforce ages, work limitations due to disabilities also increase. According to the March 2000 Current Population Survey, 6.7 percent of those aged twenty-five to thirty-four reported a work limitation. For those aged forty-five to fifty-four, the number doing so rose to nearly one in ten (9.8%), and it was 16.1 percent of those aged fifty-five to sixty-one (Burkhauser and Houtenville, in press). The rise in work limitations, coupled with a rapidly growing population of older workers, greatly increases the number of people who may require assistance from rehabilitation professionals.

The Aging U.S. Labor Force

According to U.S. Bureau of the Census population projections, by 2010 people aged forty-five to sixty-four will account for 44 percent of the working-age population. Recent changes in the Social Security system may further increase the number of older workers. Beginning in 2003, the age for receiving full Social Security benefits will gradually increase from sixty-five to sixty-seven. In addition, the earnings limit for Social Security beneficiaries aged sixty-five to sixty-nine was repealed as of March 2000. Both of these changes make it likely that individuals will remain in the workforce longer.

Employers are aware of this trend and are concerned about managing this aging labor force effectively (Elliott 1995; Lofgren 1999; Minter 2000; William M. Mercer Inc. 2000). The challenges represented by the changing labor force include addressing its members' psychosocial characteristics and their health and functioning. Silverstone (1996) suggested that this group will redefine old age and aging, moving us toward functional rather than chronological markers for what it means to be aging. In addition, the human resources literature has begun to encourage practitioners and occupational health and safety professionals to think about how to structure environments and encourage workplace practices that will reduce danger to older workers, who may be at greater risk of work-related injuries.

Statistics on Aging Workers with Disabilities

There is little information available on how aging affects the employment of workers who are already disabled. This area needs continued research with longitudinal studies. However, we do know that workers with disabilities are subject to the same declines that all people experience with age. This "functional decline" involves a decrease in strength and endurance, slower reaction time, and increase in chronic conditions such as arthritis and visual and hearing impairments that can affect work performance. It has also been reported that this type of decline in function may occur earlier or be more severe in workers with a disability than in nondisabled workers (Campbell 1999; Kemp 1999; McNeal, Somerville, and Wilson 1999). Zarb (1993) described this commonly experienced downturn in health and physical well-being as typically occurring twenty to thirty years after the onset of a disability — *independent* of the individual's chronological age. Many of these changes may be due to the long-term effects of the original disability as well as secondary impairments or long-term effects of medical interventions. According to Zarb (1993, 34), different disabilities appear to have different long-term "trajectories" as well. For example:

- progressive deterioration since onset (e.g., "burnout" in multiple sclerosis and arthritis);
- onset of gradual deterioration after twenty or more years of relative stability (spinal injuries, polio, long-term diabetes);
- onset of increasingly progressive deterioration after either a period of relative stability or only gradual deterioration (appears to be characteristic of long-term scoliosis);· intermittent change with an underlying pattern of gradually progressive deterioration (seen in Parkinson disease and multiple sclerosis).

These changes and the differences individuals with disabilities experience as they age must be understood so appropriate actions can be taken to maintain their employment.

The percentage of people with disabilities who are employed decreases for those with functional limitations, defined as difficulty in performing specific activities such as reading newspaper print, hearing normal conversation, having speech be understood, lifting or carrying ten pounds, and walking a quarter of a mile or climbing a flight of stairs without resting. Only 32 percent of people with such functional limitations are employed, compared with 82 percent of people without disabilities (Stoddard et al. 1998).

A study of the 1986 and 1991 Canadian Health and Activity Limitations Survey data (Raina et al. 2000) determined that hearing and visual impairments were the third and fourth most prevalent types of disability, respectively, among adults fifty-five and older. One in ten respondents aged fifty-five to sixty-four reported difficulty either in hearing a conversation (7.5 percent) even when using a hearing aid (with one person or in a group of three or more) or in reading normal newsprint or seeing faces from a distance (2.2 percent), even with corrective lenses. An additional 0.7 percent reported problems with both vision and hearing. The proportion experiencing such difficulties increases rapidly with age. Clearly, any one of these problems would have a significant impact on work performance and workplace communication.

A study conducted at the University of California, San Francisco, based on statistics from the Current Population Survey of 1993 conducted by the U.S. Bureau of the Census reported that during the period studied people with disabilities were more than three times as likely to leave jobs as those without disabilities. The study also reported that a high percentage of people thirty-five or older with disabilities left jobs sooner than their nondisabled counterparts. This percentage increased for disabled workers between fifty-five and sixty-four. The study concluded that a person with a disability who was lucky enough to be employed would be less likely to keep working while aging than a person without a disability (Yelin and Trupin 1997).

A longitudinal study by Grundy and Glaser (2000) examined the onset and progression of disability in early old age of a representative sample of 3,543 older adults in the United Kingdom in 1988-89 and again five years later. Of individuals aged fifty-five to fifty-nine who said they had a disability at the first survey, 31 percent rated the disability as worse in the follow-up (60 percent rated it the same, 10 percent rated it as improved). Of those aged fifty-five to fifty-nine who had not noted a disability in the first survey, 29 percent reported the onset of a disability in the follow-up five years later.

Employer Experience with Accommodations

Methodology and Sampling for Cornell University Research

For the past four years, Cornell University has been involved in research that examines the responses of both private-sector and federal employers to the employment provisions of the Americans with Disabilities Act (ADA) of 1990.[1] The ADA prohibits discrimination in all phases of employment, including hiring, promotions and transfer, training, compensation and fringe benefits, and layoffs and terminations. The research has been based on the premise that implementing the employment provisions of this legislation falls largely in the realm of human resources (HR) professionals who are responsible for recruitment, preemployment screening, and other workplace practices that affect the hiring and retention of workers with and without disabilities. The purpose of the private-sector research has been to identify how HR professionals have responded to the ADA and thereby to learn what more can be done to support their critical role in minimizing workplace discrimination for people with disabilities. The purpose was similar in the federal sector, with the added advantage of examining a workplace that has had nondiscrimination coverage for a longer time (since passage of the Rehabilitation Act of 1973).

The Survey Instruments

Two ten-page parallel surveys were developed, covering the employment provisions of the Americans with Disabilities Act of 1990 (ADA) and the Rehabilitation Act of 1973 as amended for federal organizations. The private-sector sample was a random sampling (stratified by organizational size) of the membership of the Society for Human Resource Management (SHRM) and the entire membership of the Washington Business Group on Health (WBGH). The federal agency sample included the human resources and equal employment opportunity (EEO) personnel from all ninety-seven U.S. federal agencies. Among the issues addressed were the reasonable accommodation process; recruitment, preemployment screening, testing, and new employee orientation of workers with disabilities. Response rates to the surveys were as follows: 73 percent (a total of 813 participants) of the eligible SHRM respondents, 32 percent of the WBGH membership (52 participants), and 97 percent of the federal agency respondents (403 participants).

Characteristics of Respondents

Nearly two out of five of the private-sector respondents were in service industries, another quarter were from the manufacturing sector, an additional 9 percent were in finance, and 8 percent were in high tech/computer/telecommunication industries. Two-thirds of the private-sector respondents reported their function as "HR generalist," and 8 percent reported EEO/affirmative action. Federal respondents were more evenly split between these functions (42 percent and 35 percent, respectively). Approximately seven out of ten of the private-sector respondents reported their tenure with their company as ten or fewer years, while the majority (59 percent) of the federal respondents had been with the government more than ten years. Many private-sector respondents were small employers, with 40 percent reporting fewer than 250 employees (compared with 21 percent of the federal respondents). Federal respondents tended to have more employees, with 27 percent reporting 1,500 to 4,999 employees and 23 percent reporting 5,000 or more (13 percent and 14 percent, respectively, for the private-sector respondents).

Accommodations Most Often Made

As shown in table 8.1, private-sector organizations are responding to the ADA by making accommodations for applicants and employees with disabilities. Across eleven areas where accommodation could be made, survey respondents most commonly reported making existing facilities accessible, being flexible in applying HR policies, and restructuring jobs and work hours. Other often-made changes were modifying the work environment and making transportation accommodations. Accommodations were least often made in the areas of modifying training materials and changing supervisory methods.

There was a statistically significant difference in the groups' responses to making these changes across all of the eleven categories, with federal agencies more likely to have made each change. Private-sector organizations were also more likely than federal agencies to say they had never been asked to make the changes.

Areas Found Most Difficult to Accommodate

Those surveyed were asked about their response to making changes in recruitment, preemployment screening, testing, and orientation to comply with the ADA and about how hard it was to make these changes. Across these ten screening, testing, and orientation processes where changes might have been made, 10-60 percent of all organizations reported not having needed to make these changes. Of those who did make changes in response to the ADA, most

Table 8.1. Accommodations by federal and/or private employers

Accommodation	Federal		Private	
	Accommodated	Not able to make accommodation	Accommodated	Not able to make accommodation
Acquired/modified materials	53	1	31	1
Provided qualified readers/interpreters	80	0	36	0
Changed supervisory methods	64	0	36	2
Made reassignment to vacant positions	62	2	47	1
Acquired/modified equipment or devices	92	0	59	0
Modified work environment	93	0	63	0
Provided written job instructions	76	0	65	0
Made parking or transportation accommodations	87	2	67	0
Restructured jobs or modified work hours	88	1	69	0
Were flexible with policies on work hours	96	0	80	0
Made existing facilities accessible	94	0	82	1

said they were relatively easy to make (table 8.2). Respondents in both sectors said it was hard to make information accessible to people with visual, learning, or hearing impairments. There was a statistically significant difference between sectors in their response in three of the ten categories for accommodation. Private-sector respondents reported more difficulty in making information accessible to people with visual impairments (36 percent compared with 15 percent for federal respondents), and private-sector employers reported more difficulty in making information accessible to people with hearing im-

Table 8.2. Ease of making preemployment accommodations by federal and private employers (of those who made changes)

Accommodation	Percentage rating change easy	
	Federal	Private
Employee orientation accessible	89	85
Medical test after offer	75	75
Interview locations accessible	85	80
Recruiting locations accessible	76	74
Changing wording of job application	84	75
Changing interview questions	78	72
Modifying preemployment testing	69	67
Restroom accessible	76	73
Information for hearing impaired	77	49
Information for visually or learning impaired	64	35

pairments (25 percent and 8 percent, for private-sector and federal respondents, respectively). Federal agency representatives expressed less difficulty in every listed change except one: providing medical tests after a job offer was made. It might be interesting to explore whether federal organizations' perception of these accommodations as being less difficult comes from their having had more time under these requirements as a function of the Rehabilitation Act of 1973.

Implications for an Aging Workforce with Disabilities

It is interesting that human resources professionals interviewed in this study said they were less familiar with accommodations for people with hearing and vision impairments than with accommodations of other kinds. Respondents were presented with a number of ADA compliance considerations in interviewing applicants and asked how familiar their organizations' interview staff was with each of these elements. In general, respondents reported the highest levels of familiarity with framing questions about job tasks, when to ask how the applicant would perform job tasks, and restrictions on obtaining medical information. Across groups, respondents were much less familiar with accommodations for people with visual or hearing impairments, such as adapting print materials or providing a reader for people with visual impairments and using TTY/text telephones to set up interviews. Federal respondents indicated a much greater familiarity with accessing sign-language interpreters (33 percent of private sector compared with 76 percent of federal respondents reported their staff was "familiar" or "very familiar" with this issue). Federal respondents, while least familiar with accommodations for vision or hearing impairments, were far more familiar with them than their private-sector counterparts. The private-sector and federal respondents showed statistically significant differences in their responses in five of the eight ADA compliance considerations presented.

Since diminution of hearing and visual acuity is a natural part of aging for all of us, it seems imperative that employers begin to acquire the needed problem-solving skills and information to deal with these issues effectively.

Perceived Barriers and Preferred Employer Intervention Strategies

Respondents were presented with seven possible barriers to the employment and advancement of people with disabilities. In general, the profile of perceived barriers, in terms of overall percentage of responses, was similar in both the private and the federal groups. Interestingly, in both the federal and the private sectors, increased costs—of training, supervision, and accommodations for applicants or employees with disabilities—were least likely to be rated as significant continuing barriers compared with other areas. The largest continuing barriers to employment and advancement for people with disabilities reported by both federal and private-sector employers were their lack of related experience (49 percent reported by private sector and 53 percent by federal) and their lack of requisite skills and training (39 percent for private-sector respondents and 45 percent for federal). The next most often cited was supervisors' knowledge of how to make accommodations (31 percent in the private-sector group and 34 percent in the federal). Stereotypes or poor attitudes among coworkers and supervisors toward people with disabilities were seen as the third most significant barrier among federal respondents (43 percent) and fifth among private-sector respondents (22 percent).

Respondents were also asked to rate the effectiveness of six specific ways of reducing these barriers. The top way identified by both sectors was the same: a visible top management commitment (81 percent for the private-sector respondents, 90 percent for federal). This is therefore very important information for rehabilitation providers providing workplace interventions. The next three ways were staff training (62 percent of private sector and 71 percent of federal), mentoring (59 percent and 71 percent), and on-site consultation or technical assistance (58 percent and 71 percent). Tax incentives were seen as the least effective way to reduce such barriers by private-sector employers— only 26 percent reported these as effective or very effective in reducing barriers. A parallel item regarding special budget allocations as a way to reduce accommodation costs to employers was asked on the federal survey. Sixty-nine percent of those interviewed saw this as effective or very effective in reducing barriers.

The Role of Vocational Rehabilitation Service Providers

Legislation such as the ADA presents an additional tool for rehabilitation professionals to use when working with employers in the areas of job development and job placement for people with disabilities. Although similar protections were in place with the Rehabilitation Act of 1993 under Title V, the ADA extends this coverage to all employers of fifteen employees or more and thereby greatly broadens regulatory disability nondiscrimination influence on employer policies and practices.

Under the ADA employment provisions, employers are not required to provide specific accommodations for a particular disability. Instead, they are encouraged to engage in informal problem solving with the individual applicant or employee to identify the appropriate accommodation. Each individual with a disability is seen as unique; therefore every opportunity to address a barrier to employment needs to be considered relative to the situation. Rehabilitation personnel can make a significant contribution by working closely with employers, the employees, and other professionals in the workplace. As employees with disabilities experience changes in function at work as a result of aging, knowledgeable vocational practitioners and therapists can help them keep their jobs by being available to find ways to accommodate these changes.

The results of the Cornell University research suggest that employers are making accommodations, but that they have less experience with some particular ones and find them more difficult, such as those for individuals with vision or hearing impairment or loss. The research results indicate that employers see certain interventions or strategies as most effective in addressing the disability issues in the workplace. Vocational rehabilitation practitioners (including vocational rehabilitation counselors, therapists, and disability management specialists) should equip themselves to contribute to such perceived effective interventions as engendering top management support for hiring and retaining workers with disabilities. In addition, since training, mentoring, and on-site consultation and assistance are seen as advantageous intervention strategies, rehabilitation practitioners should be prepared to offer these services to employers as disability questions arise.

Accommodating Workers Aging with Disabilities

The Cornell study focused on what employers had done in response to the employment provisions in disability employment nondiscrimination legislation. A study at the Rehabilitation Research and Training Center (RRTC) on Aging with a Disability at Rancho Los Amigos National Rehabilitation Center looked at accommodating aging workers who have disabilities from the workers' perspective. Two disability groups were studied, consisting of fifty individuals with postpolio and forty-six with spinal cord injury (SCI). To be eligible to participate, the individuals had to have worked twenty or more hours per week for at least five years since the onset of their disability or be retired for less than five years before the time of the study.

Most of the participants for the study were recruited from a shared database at the RRTC on Aging with a Disability. Additional participants were recruited through community contacts. Data were collected through telephone interviews that took between forty-five and ninety minutes. The interviews focused on whether employees who were aging with their disability had experienced new work problems as a consequence of functional declines and whether their work problems were accommodated.

Slightly more than one-third of the employees in the Rancho Los Amigos study said yes when asked if functional decline had interfered with continuing ability to do their jobs. In the group of employees with polio, respondents stated that their daily lives were affected by the functional decline they had experienced since their original illness. In addition, forty-one of the fifty participants in the group rated their disability as more severe at the time of the interview than when they first began their jobs. They reported that most of the work problems they identified would have been less troublesome given their physical abilities when they first began working.

Only one-third of the employees with SCI reported additional functional declines since their injury that interfered with their work. Most interviewees stated that their current problems would have been as troublesome when they first started working as when the interview was conducted. The individuals in the SCI sample were relatively younger (forty-two, on average), which may explain why their results did not conclusively show that aging with an SCI resulted in functional declines that could interfere with work. However, data from other studies suggest that as these individuals age, they experience pain in upper extremity joints and muscles, skin breakdown, and chronic urinary tract infections (Corbett 1993; Reynolds 1993). Other researchers think we can anticipate that many vital work-related activities such as parking, building access, and lifting will become difficult for individuals with SCI as they age and that some of the problems may be proactively resolved by accommodation (Gerhart et al. 1993; McNeal, Somerville, and Wilson 1999).

Typical Work Problems

The categories of problems most commonly reported by the employees were difficulty with using equipment, tools, and furniture; accessing the work site; performing specific job tasks (e.g., lifting, carrying); performing or obtaining assistance for personal care; and transportation (table 8.3). The largest number of problems experienced by the group with polio fell into the category of access to the job and included reported difficulty with climbing stairs and walking long distances from parking areas or inside the workplace. Other problems were equally distributed between categories of using equipment/tools/furniture; lifting, carrying, or moving items needed to perform specific job tasks; and a category labeled "getting the job done," which included the effect on productivity of the muscle weakness, fatigue, and pain experienced by most employees in this group.

The SCI group had the largest number of problems in the category of using equipment/tools/furniture. More than a third of the problems reported in this category were related to inability to reach the desk or items on the desk from a wheelchair. Other problems included in this category involved using computers, telephones, and file cabinets and loading paper into printers, copiers, and fax machines. The second largest number of problems for this disability group were in the category of access. These problems included having to wheel manual wheelchairs long distances from parking sites or inside the work site. These employees complained about not being able to get to the entrances or interior areas because of stairs or about inability to open heavy doors or use a

Table 8.3. Types of work problem identified by study participants (%)

Problem category	Type of problem included	Report by disability	
		Polio	SCI
Using equipment/tools/ furniture	Computer/typewriters Telephones Office furniture Equipment/tools/furniture not used in offices	21.3	39
Access	To parking To and within work site To restrooms	30.8	24.3
Getting the job done	Working a fixed schedule Reduced productivity Getting job done, but fatigued	16.3	10.8
Performing tasks	Lifting/carrying/pushing/pulling Standing/walking/climbing Other tasks	20.4	9.7
Personal care	Eating/drinking Toileting Commuting/local travel Travel	1.4	8.1
Other		4.1	0.8

keycard. A number of employees expressed a need for flexible work schedules because they had trouble getting to work on time or needed time off for medical appointments or personal care.

Employees tended to underreport the number of work-related problems they were experiencing, as verified by a small number of work-site evaluations completed for self-selected employees. One reason for understatement of problems is that employees were used to doing tasks a certain way and to using available tools, equipment, and furniture and were slow to recognize when these were no longer effective. Another reason is that many employees thought there was no way to solve specific problems and so had just learned to live with them.

Accommodating Work Problems

The employees in the Rancho Los Amigos study worked primarily for large private organizations that employed more than two hundred people. The accommodations they most frequently used were special equipment, furniture, and tools or modification of standard items; assistance from coworkers; modification of job tasks or procedures; architectural modifications; and changing employee behavior on the job (table 8.4). The employees felt that accommodation was vital to maintaining their employment. One-third of those who received accommodations stated that they could not have continued to work without them. However, it was found that many of these accommodations were not satisfactory to the employees. Slightly more than half of the problems experienced by the polio group and just over two-thirds of those experienced by the SCI group were considered to have satisfactory solutions. Problems not accommodated or not satisfactorily accommodated were found to affect both the work and the personal lives of the employees with disabilities. Often their personal lives were affected first, with participants making changes in activities of daily living or lifestyle changes to conserve energy for work. Work was eventually affected in a variety of ways, including absences, lower productivity, job changes, working fewer hours per day or fewer days per week, or working a more flexible schedule. Providing a satisfactory accommodation allows people to perform tasks that were otherwise difficult and to do them with less stress and fatigue.

Most employees in both the polio and SCI groups were not aware of the resources available outside the work site to help them solve work problems. Less than 10 percent of the accommodations received were obtained through outside resources such as vocational rehabilitation agencies, technology experts, vendors, or information databases. The vast majority were obtained by talking to employers or coworkers or made by employees on their own behalf. Most of the problems that did not have a satisfactory resolution had no accommodation identified. This fact, coupled with the report that sources outside the companies were consulted in only 10 percent of the cases, confirms the lack of knowledge and use of available resources.

Employer Considerations

Employers did not usually refuse employees' requests for accommodations. Only 18 out of a total of 480 problems for both groups were not accommo-

Table 8.4. Accommodations provided for problem categories (%)

		Report by disability	
Accommodation category	Accommodation	Polio	SCI
Equipment / furniture / tools		29.0	45.1
	Purchase standard items		
	Purchase special items		
	Modify standard items		
Assistance from others		21.5	25.2
	Coworker assistance		
	Paid assistance		
	Family assistance		
Job process modifications		17.2	11.8
	Flexible schedule		
	Reduced hours		
	Modify/eliminate tasks		
	Work at home		
Architectural modifications		14.0	10.8
	Structural		
	Environmental		
	Signage/parking permits		
	Rearrange		
	Funiture/materials		
Changed behavior		12.4	3.3
	ADL change		
	Conservation/pacing		
Other		5.9	3.9

dated because the employer refused. The employees in the Rancho Los Amigos study were reluctant to ask their employers for accommodations. This reluctance on their part may help to explain Cornell's finding that employers commonly responded "no, never needed to make [a particular] accommodation." The polio group stated that their reasons for not asking included their thinking that the accommodation needed would be too costly, that they should wait for a more opportune time to ask, or that the problem was not important enough. Many of these participants did not want to "call attention" to their disability in the workplace and were willing to try to work around the problem. Although the SCI group asked for accommodations more frequently, they did not ask their employers for accommodation for thirty-three reported problems, frequently citing the same reasons as the polio group.

Cost was not as much a factor in receiving accommodations as the employees' failure to ask. The average cost of the accommodations reported by employees in the Rancho Los Amigos study agreed with the survey of large companies completed in 1982 by Berkeley Planning Associates. Fifty-one percent of the accommodations provided cost nothing, and 80 percent cost $500 or less. More recent data from the Job Accommodation Network continue to bear out this cost of accommodation figure.[2] The $500 does not appear to be a significant deterrent to providing accommodations by very large employers, but it could be a "big deal" for a smaller company, especially if outside sources for assistance is not used. However, fewer than 25 percent of even the smallest employers surveyed in the Cornell study saw accommodation costs as a barrier to employment or advancement for people with disabilities. There appears to be a disconnection between employee and employer perceptions on the issue of accommodation costs.

In the Rancho Los Amigos study, employers paid for most of the accommodations provided. The employees paid for 22 percent of their accommodations. Private and public insurance paid for only 4 percent of the accommodations for employees in the polio group and 5.2 percent for individuals with SCI. The California Department of Rehabilitation paid for 16.8 percent of the accommodations for employees with SCI but none of the accommodations used by employees with postpolio syndrome. Again, this emphasizes the lack of knowledge of available resources for assistance.

When employees were asked to describe the attitude of their employers, supervisors, and coworkers toward their need for accommodation, most said their company, supervisor, and coworkers were supportive. However, even though the responses indicated positive attitudes among current supervisors, many employees did report that they had had supervisors with negative attitudes earlier in their work history.

Implications for Rehabilitation Therapists

As data increase to substantiate that accommodation needs change as workers with disabilities age, some major adjustments will be required in how rehabilitation therapists address functional problems when people with disabilities are young or first disabled. The focus of these therapists is currently on acute problems and the assistive technology needed to make people independent initially. This focus may be short-sighted. What may be an adequate solution for a twenty-year-old with SCI in the first five years after injury may not address the needs of that person at age forty. As technology improves and more solutions for functional problems are available, therapists need to make their recommendations in such a way that the solutions can change with the individual. We have done this for years with our pediatric population by taking growth and development into consideration for all of our strategies and recommendations. We now need to adapt these same principles to individuals who are aging with their disability. We need to educate these individuals and prepare them for functional changes and the impact of these changes on their lives at home or work. We also have an obligation to educate insurers, case managers, counselors, employers, and teachers about the changing needs that may occur owing to aging with a disability. Long-term goals should no longer stop with maximum independence in current activities of daily living but should be written to allow independence throughout the life span (Corbett 1993; Reynolds 1993). If a person with an SCI is prescribed a manual, lightweight wheelchair at age twenty, he and his insurers, parents, and any significant others need to know that the replacement chair at age thirty-five or forty should most likely be powered. If a person with postpolio at age thirty can walk to inspect facilities in his job as a real estate surveyor, he and his insurers and significant others need to know that a wheelchair or powered scooter may be needed to help him keep his job at age forty or fifty.

Therapists are also obligated to analyze the methods people use to accomplish tasks in order to teach the most energy-efficient method and to encourage the use of appropriate assistive technology. This may reduce the number of repetitive motion injuries, decrease pain and fatigue from overuse, and alleviate joint limitations that a population aging with a disability will suffer. The rehabilitation culture has always valued "hard work" as a means for individuals with disabilities to maintain strength and joint mobility. In our zeal we frequently recommend functional solutions that perhaps require more work than the therapists themselves would be willing to do in the same circumstances. One example is encouraging a person with tetraplegia to dress himself, even if it takes more than an hour and a half. Perhaps it would be better to help him get aid to dress so as to save energy for work or leisure tasks that add more to the quality of life. There are many other examples, but the principle remains the same. Rehabilitation therapists need to adjust their thinking to consider the result of functional decline on the long-term performance of tasks and its effect on the future independence of people aging with disabilities.

Summary

Statistics about the aging workforce substantiate the need for both employers and professionals who support the workforce to be prepared to deal with the unique considerations of people aging with disabilities. This chapter has discussed two studies, conducted independently by Cornell University and Rancho Los Amigos National Rehabilitation Center, that provide information on the workplace and people with disabilities. Both studies show that most employers make accommodations when asked (more than 95 percent). However, the Rancho Los Amigos study shows that individuals with disabilities were reluctant to ask for further accommodations, and Cornell's results suggest the same result from the employers' perspective, with many reporting that they "never needed to make" specific accommodations. Rehabilitation professionals could work with employers to simplify and ease the process of making accommodation requests so it is less threatening to employees and works better for all involved.

One of the concerns noted by the employees with disabilities in the Rancho Los Amigos study was their comfort level with requesting accommodations. That study suggests that employees tend to delay making changes or requesting accommodations until the difficulty is more significant and is causing further problems. Rehabilitation professionals and therapists should have a place in working as mediators/communicators between employees with disabilities and employers to provide proactive accommodations. This would have a great impact on the quality of work life for employees with disabilities as well as on their personal life (which tends to be affected first, according to the Rancho Los Amigos study).

There is a need to educate both employers and the employees about changes in limitations that can occur as people with disabilities age. Rehabilitation professionals and therapists may be able to inform both groups about the possible courses of aging with particular disabilities and to work with them to determine the best way to deal with the difficulties and new challenges these changes produce.

In addition, they can work with both employees and employers to develop better strategies or accommodations (since many employees were dissatisfied with accommodations that had been made). As the Rancho Los Amigos study found, even the employees themselves tend to underreport the number of work-related problems they are experiencing. They are not always aware of problems on the work site and often just live with them. Rehabilitation professionals and therapists can perhaps reanalyze to see if new issues emerge as an employee with a disability ages.

Rehabilitation professionals can also assist both the employer and employees by pointing out both the internal and the community resources available to help with the issues of an aging workforce. Results from the Cornell study suggest that employers that have a return-to-work or disability management program believe it is helpful with several issues of accommodation as well as making supervisors and coworkers more aware and accepting of employees with disabilities. Developing such a program can promote ready accommodations as well as creating a more receptive climate for a workforce whose members are aging and may also have disabilities. In addition, it may be important to educate employers and employees on sources of assistance outside the workplace, such as job coaching, matching funds for specific accommodations, and professionals who can address specific needs. These may well provide more satisfactory ways (or at least a greater universe of possibilities) to generate accommodations appropriate and satisfactory to the individual with the disability.

Because studies have shown that people with disabilities are more likely to remain employed if they are accommodated, rehabilitation professionals can be invaluable in helping employers retain valued and experienced employees, thereby saving them money on hiring and training new employees. Such contributions by rehabilitation professionals and therapists may well extend beyond working just with those with disabilities. As the Cornell study pointed out, accommodations related to hearing and vision impairments are some of the ones least understood by employers yet most needed as the workforce ages. Addressing the impairments of workers with disabilities can help the broader aging workforce as well.

NOTES

1. The U.S. Department of Education National Institute on Disability and Rehabilitation Research sponsored the Cornell research in the private sector (Grant no. H133A70005); the Presidential Task Force on Employment of Adults with Disabilities sponsored the study of the federal sector by Cornell University.

2. The Job Accommodation Network (JAN) is an international toll-free consulting ser-

vice that provides information about job accommodations and the employability of people with disabilities; it can be found on the Web at http://janweb.icdi.wvu.edu/.

REFERENCES

Berkeley Planning Associates. 1982. *A study of accommodations provided to handicapped employees by federal contractors.* Final Report, vol. 1, *Study findings.* Berkeley, Calif.: Berkeley Planning Associates.

Burkhauser, R. V., and Houtenville, A. J. In press. Employment among working-age people with disabilities: What current data can tell us. In *Work and disability: Issues and strategies for career development and job placement,* ed. E. M. Szymanski and R. M. Parker, 2nd ed. Austin, Tex.: Pro-Ed.

Campbell, M. L. 1999. Secondary conditions experienced by persons aging with long-term physical disability: Scope and implications for assistive technology and other services. Paper presented at RESNA's Fifth Annual Research Symposium, Long Beach, Calif.

Corbett, B. 1993. What price independence? In *Aging with spinal cord injury,* ed. K. Gerhart, S. Charlifue, R. Menter, D. Weitzenkamp, and G. Whiteneck, 229–38. New York: Demos Medical Publishing.

Elliott, R. 1995. Human resource management's role in the future aging of the workforce. *Review of Public Personnel Administration* 15 (2): 5–17.

Gerhart, K., Charlifue, S., Menter, R., Weitzenkamp, D., and Whiteneck, G., eds. 1993. *Aging with spinal cord injury.* New York: Demos Medical Publishing.

Grundy, E., and Glaser, K. 2000. Socio-demographic differences in the onset and progression of disability in early old age: A longitudinal study. *Age and Ageing* 29:149–57.

Kemp, B. 1999. Aging with a disability: What's been learned? *New Mobility,* April 1999, 28–34.

Lofgren, E. 1999. Workforce management is new discipline for the future. *Compensation and Benefits Management* 15 (1): 13–18.

McNeal, D. R., Somerville, N., and Wilson, D. 1999. Work problems and accommodations reported by persons who are post polio or have a spinal cord injury. *Assistive Technology* 11:137–57.

Minter, S. 2000. Keeping older workers safe and productive. *Occupational Hazards* 62 (11): 6.

Raina, P., Wong, M., Dukeshire, S., Chambers, L., and Lindsay, J. 2000. Prevalence, risk factors, and self reported medical causes of seeing and hearing-related disabilities among older adults. *Canadian Journal on Aging* 19 (2): 260–78.

Reynolds, G. R. 1993. Becoming successful health care consumers. In *Aging with spinal cord injury,* ed. K. Gerhart., S. Charlifue, R. Menter, D. Weitzenkamp, and G. Whiteneck, 229-38. New York: Demos Medical Publishing.

Silverstone, B. 1996. Older people of tomorrow: A psychosocial profile. *Gerontologist* 36 (1): 27–32.

Stoddard, S., Jans, L., Ripple, J. M., and Kraus, L. 1998. *Chartbook on work and disability in the United States.* Prepared under Grant no. H133D50017-96 from the U.S. Department of Education, National Institute on Disability and Rehabilitation Research. Washington, D.C.: U.S. Department of Education, National Institute on Disability and Rehabilitation Research.

U.S. Bureau of the Census. 2000. *Current population survey 2000.* Washington, D.C.: U.S. Department of Commerce.

William M. Mercer Inc. 2000. *Capitalizing on an aging workforce.* New York: William M. Mercer.

Yelin, E., and Trupin, L. 1997. Successful labor market transitions for persons with disabilities: Factors affecting the probability of entering and maintaining employment. Paper prepared for Conference on Employment Post the Americans with Disabilities Act. Sponsored by Office of Disability, Social Security Administration, and National Institute on Disability and Rehabilitation Research, Washington, D.C.

Zarb, G. 1993. "Forgotten but not gone": The experience of aging with a disability. In *Aging, independence and the life course,* ed. S. Aber and M. J. Evandrou. London: Kingsley.

Part 4

Impairment-Specific Conditions

9

Aging with a Spinal Cord Injury

William A. Bauman, M.D., and Robert L. Waters, M.D.

Spinal cord injury (SCI) typically occurs in young males and is often due to high-speed vehicular trauma or, increasingly, violence. The incidence of SCI in the United States is approximately 10,000 cases per year, with a prevalence of 200,000 cases. Damage to the spinal cord is categorized by level of injury (paraplegia or tetraplegia) and by severity of injury (complete or incomplete). The International Standards for Neurological and Functional Classification of SCI are used to assess motor and sensory function as well as completeness of injury (ASIA/IMSOP 1996). These standards represent the most valid and reliable data set for assessing SCI.

Within the past five decades, long-term survival of people with SCI has improved dramatically. Categorical treatment programs for SCI, which were established during and shortly after World War II, and the introduction of antibiotics and specialized urologic management have dramatically increased life expectancy. Life expectancy, however, still remains slightly below normal, and people with greater neurological deficits tend to die earlier. Mortality is highest in the first year after the injury, but life expectancy increases significantly for those who survive the first year.

Previously, the major causes of death for individuals with SCI were renal failure and urinary tract complications. Improvements in the management of the neurogenic bladder and prevention of renal failure have significantly decreased urinary tract complications and the associated mortality and morbidity. The most recent studies of mortality have identified respiratory system complications, cardiovascular conditions, and external events (suicide, homicide, accidents) as major causes of death after the initial year following injury.

As life expectancy for those with SCI approaches that for able-bodied people, aging with an SCI has become an increasingly significant concern for patients and a key research issue. Patients are concerned with the quality of their remaining years. Clinicians are specifically concerned with preserving function and with identifying the issues of aging that are now presenting themselves in the SCI population. Among the questions researchers are attempting to answer are: Are the pattern and onset of aging different (more adverse) for people with SCI? What are the aging changes specific to particular organ systems? Are there interventions that can successfully minimize the potential effect of aging with SCI?

Researchers are in general agreement that those with SCI demonstrate atypical aging. That is, medical and functional changes associated with aging occur at an earlier age than they do in the able-bodied population, and SCI-specific aging changes are attributed to the unique physical characteristics of this population. In this chapter we will present the most significant aspect of aging with SCI for the various body systems.

Skin

People with SCI are at risk for pressure ulcers owing to immobility, diminished or absent sensation, and spasticity. People with intact motor and sensory functions reposition themselves unconsciously throughout the day and night to prevent excess unrelieved pressure over any one area. Those with impaired sensation and motor function cannot do this and must make a conscious effort to avoid pressure buildup.

The risk of developing pressure sores has been demonstrated to increase with the time since injury: 15 percent at one year after the injury, 30 percent at twenty years after the injury (Consortium for Spinal Cord Medicine 2000). Age also affects the development of pressure ulcers, since aging skin is less resistant to shearing forces and more susceptible to pressure ulcers. As a result, sitting and turning tolerances may decrease.

The primary means of preventing pressure sores is through patient education (Nash and Fletcher 1993). Patients are taught techniques of skin inspection, pressure relief, and positioning. They must be vigilant in inspecting their skin for any redness that does not resolve within an hour, temperature changes ("hot spots" or "cold spots"), and edema. Pressure relief is accomplished by arm raises, weight shifting, or positioning in the wheelchair. People who are independent in arm raises should perform them for fifteen seconds every fifteen minutes. Those who need help should perform pressure relief for one minute every hour. Sleeping in the prone position or turning every two hours has been shown to prevent pressure ulcers. Sitting tolerance must be closely monitored, and sitting time must be reduced if there are signs of excess pressure. Typically, sitting tolerance is limited to thirty to sixty minutes initially. If redness resolves within thirty minutes, sitting time can be gradually increased. Sitting tolerance may decrease after prolonged periods of bed rest, after hospitalization, or after trauma to a weight-bearing area.

Various mechanical aids such as specialized wheelchair cushions and mattresses may be used to minimize skin pressure. It is important that the efficacy of such equipment be regularly monitored. It is essential that patients understand that specialized equipment does not eliminate the need for basic pressure relief maneuvers but merely augments them. As patients age they may notice a decreased sitting tolerance or an increased need for pressure relief. The onset of superficial pressure sores often signals an increased susceptibility, so skin care procedures must be reevaluated and refined. Strategies to maintain skin integrity in the aging population may include more frequent pressure relief or repositioning, acceptance of decreased sitting tolerance, or use of equipment such as specialized wheelchair cushions, beds, or mattresses to augment fundamental pressure relief.

Pressure ulcers in people with SCI have been associated with increased energy requirements. In people with paraplegia, a hypermetabolic state may ensue. However, because the basal or resting metabolism of an individual with tetraplegia may be hypometabolic, a pressure ulcer may raise metabolic demands only into the normal metabolic range. Even while hospitalized for care of their pressure ulcers, people with tetraplegia have been found to use less than the normal resting energy expenditure. A significant relationship exists between the area of the pressure ulcer and the percentage increase in resting energy expenditure. Anecdotal case study reports in the literature have found that anabolic steroids may be efficacious in treating nonhealing pressure ulcers in patients receiving conventional clinical care. In patients who have weight loss and pressure ulcers that will not heal despite optimal medical and surgical care, a trial with anabolic agents may prove beneficial, although at present their therapeutic efficacy is unproved (Demling and DeSanti 1998).

Musculoskeletal

Noticeable aging changes in the musculoskeletal system in the nondisabled population generally begin in early adulthood, usually in the third decade. These changes include decreased muscular strength; decreased flexibility of soft tissues such as skin, joint capsules, ligaments, and tendons; and decreased shock absorption and joint lubrication (Waters, Sie, and Adkins 2001). Osteoarthritis, which can be classified as primary or secondary, typically occurs in the weight-bearing joints. Primary osteoarthritis is the exacerbation of normal aging, while secondary osteoarthritis occurs as a response to trauma or deformity. Changes in the joint surface alter the biomechanics of the joint. Continued use of the joint will worsen degeneration and accompanying signs and symptoms, such as pain, tenderness, deformity, and decreased range of motion.

Immobilization Osteoporosis and Calcium Metabolism

SCI produces immediate and permanent unloading of the gravity-bearing skeletal regions. Acute immobilization causes skeletal structural and metabolic changes. Urinary calcium excretion increases within days, reaching a maximum between one and six months after injury. Elevation of serum calcium can occur in adults with acute SCI when bone resorption is increased in association with an impaired fractional excretion of calcium by the kidney. Symptoms of immobilization hypercalcemia usually develop relatively early after SCI, weeks to months after acute injury. Hypercalcemia should be in the differential diagnosis of any patient with acute or subacute SCI who experiences nausea, vomiting, anorexia, fatigue, lethargy, polydipsia, polyuria, or dehydration. Risk factors for hypercalcemia include recent paralysis, male gender, complete neurological injuries, high cervical injury, dehydration, and prolonged immobilization. The maximum urinary calcium in those with SCI is two to four times that of able-bodied subjects who were voluntarily placed on prolonged bed rest. Calciuria has not been shown to be reduced by passive weight-bearing exercise or wheelchair activity. After acute SCI, the parathyroid hormone–vitamin D axis is suppressed. Although urinary calcium was markedly elevated on a low calcium diet, increasing dietary calcium in a subset of patients with acute SCI did not further raise either urinary or serum calcium concentrations. The finding of hypercalciuria and hypercalcemia after acute SCI has led to the misguided clinical practice of restricting dietary calcium at the time of acute injury, an ineffective and unnecessary intervention.

A dramatic reduction in bone mineral content and bone mineral density has been amply documented in people with chronic SCI (Bauman, Garland, and Schwartz 1997). Osteoporosis generally involves the pelvis and lower extremities in people with paraplegia, while those with tetraplegia lose bone in the upper extremities as well. In those with incomplete SCI of the Brown-Sequard type, the mean bone density of the paretic knee was lower than that of the stronger knee, with leg strength and bone density moderately correlated. In sets of identical twins, one of whom had paraplegia, those with paraplegia had a loss of bone density in the pelvis and lower extremities compared with their twins. The depletion of bone mineral appeared to be progressive over decades after injury.

Osteoporosis and increased risk of fractures are well-established complications for people with chronic SCI (Stewart et al. 1982). Pathological fractures of the long bones occur in those with SCI after negligible stress or trauma, such as during transfer maneuvers, range of motion exercises, bending, or minor falls. Several studies have addressed lower extremity fractures in people with SCI. Attempts to improve bone mass and strength by modulating muscle tone, activity, or weight-bearing have yielded negligible benefits.

Although disuse may be the primary cause of osteopenia in people with SCI, nutritional deficiencies may contribute, particularly those involving calcium and vitamin D (Bauman, Zhong, and Schwartz 1995). Because of the tendency for calcium nephrolithiasis soon after acute SCI, people with chronic SCI are often instructed to restrict calcium intake, chiefly dairy products. This restriction may also result in vitamin D deficiency, since dairy products, especially milk, are fortified with vitamin D and generally are the main source of dietary vitamin D. Reduced calcium and vitamin D intake would be expected to worsen the bone loss of immobilization.

Upper Extremities

The upper extremities were designed for prehension, not for locomotion, weight bearing, or stabilization. In people with SCI, the upper extremities are used for achieving mobility, such as by wheelchair propulsion, as well as for weight bearing, as in transfers, pressure relief, or walking with crutches.

The ability to use the upper extremities depends on the level and severity of injury. For people with tetraplegia, function can range from independent wheelchair mobility to total dependence for all mobility and self-care. Level and severity of injury also affect the amount of upper extremity assistance required to augment lower extremity weakness in people with paraplegia.

Since those with SCI rely on their upper extremities for weight bearing and mobility as well as prehension, they are more susceptible to upper extremity impairments (Waters and Sie 2001). Furthermore, the consequences of upper extremity impairments are greater than in the able-bodied population and may result in a functional level that is worse than the actual neurological level of injury.

Shoulder pain is one of the most common complaints among people with SCI. Various investigators have documented the prevalence of shoulder pain as between 30 and 73 percent. Rotator cuff problems, capsular contracture, and anterior instability were frequently identified as the cause. Tasks most often related to shoulder pain were propelling a wheelchair up an incline, transfers, and sleeping.

Factors that precipitate overuse and degenerative change in the shoulder are rotator cuff compression and fatigue owing to repetitive or static shoulder elevation; work posture; chronological age; and compression and ischemia within the shoulder joint owing to weight bearing during wheelchair propulsion and when performing transfers (Pentland and Twomey 1994). Shoulder muscle imbalance has also been implicated in upper extremity pain.

A physician or physical therapist may advise the patient on how to modify the way wheeling, transfers, or other activities of daily living are performed to decrease shoulder stress. Ergonomic analysis of other commonly performed tasks such as overhead reaching to minimize shoulder stress can be highly beneficial in relieving pain. Substituting a powered chair for a manual chair to lessen the demand on the shoulders may be necessary when there is moderate or severe degeneration and when conservative measures such as anti-inflammatory medications, steroid injections, or exercises fail.

Lower Extremities

Degenerative changes in the lower extremities in people with SCI are less common than changes in the upper extremities. The knee is the most common site of musculoskeletal degeneration in the lower extremities. This occurs most often in people who can walk but who have gait abnormalities that generate deviant forces at the knee. People who are not ambulatory rarely, if ever, have degenerative changes. Pathological fractures, however, are a concern. Most occur in the lower extremities, with supracondylar femoral fractures, femoral shaft fractures, and tibial fractures being the most common types.

Patient education is a key factor in maintaining the functional independence of people aging with SCI. Research and development of treatment strategies will also become increasingly important as the number of people aging with SCI increases. Individuals may need to be counseled to accept modifications in their assistive devices or to accept help they did not need before. For example, they may need a powered wheelchair to preserve upper extremity function when previously they relied on a manual wheelchair. They may also need to conserve energy or to pace their activities. Additionally, it may be necessary for individuals and for society to modify their expectations of realistic long-term functional independence. It may not be prudent to try to maintain maximum function if it accelerates degenerative changes in the musculoskeletal system.

Immune System

A decline in immune system function, an increase in the incidence of infection, and greater susceptibility to autoimmune and neoplastic diseases are associated with normal aging. Other factors that are often associated with aging and that also affect immune system function include nutritional deficiency, depression, pain, loneliness, diminishing social support, and increased use of medications. Although the immune system has not been studied as much as other organ systems, evidence suggests that immune system dysfunction may accompany SCI, especially in those with tetraplegia (Nash and Fletcher 1993). As a person with SCI ages, the incidence of urinary tract infection (UTI) increases. Since people with SCI are already at a higher risk for UTI owing to indwelling urinary drainage systems, and since respiratory complications (especially pneumonia) are the leading cause of mortality for those with tetraplegia, it seems prudent to determine the course of immune system function in aging SCI survivors. When their patterns of immune function are determined, interventions may be implemented, which one hopes will improve immune defenses against respiratory, urinary tract, and other infections.

Nervous System

Decrease in vibratory sense, muscle mass, and strength as well as slower reaction times, decreased coordination, and agility are associated with aging of the nervous system. For individuals aging with SCI, common neurologic impairments also include sensory loss and progressive motor deficits. Histological examination of the spinal cord after the fifth decade reveals loss of myelinated tracts and a loss of anterior horn cells.

Entrapment neuropathies have been documented in up to 63 percent of individuals with paraplegia. The most common site is entrapment of the median nerve at the wrist (carpal tunnel syndrome). Signs and symptoms of carpal tunnel syndrome include sensory loss in the median nerve distribution, weakness of thumb abduction and opposition, and pain in the wrist and the hand. Repetitive contact of the hand with the wheelchair hand rims and increased intracanal pressures during pressure relief raises and transfers have been implicated in carpal tunnel syndrome. Modifying activities of daily living and splinting the wrists in a neutral position may alleviate symptoms. If surgical release of the transverse carpal ligament is necessary, individuals must be ready for more dependence on adaptive equipment or physical assistance during recovery. Entrapments of the ulnar nerve at the wrist and elbow have also been observed but are less common than median nerve entrapments among those with SCI. They are also typically more responsive to conservative treatment.

Approximately 5 percent of people with SCI develop neurologic deterioration after years of relative stability in function. Late-onset neurologic deterioration may be due to posttraumatic syringomyelia. In this condition there is a progressively enlarging cavity within the spinal cord that may extend downward or upward from the initial injury. Symptoms may include deterioration of motor or sensory function, increased pain, spasticity, or poor reflexes as well as hyperhidrosis and Horner syndrome. Diagnosis is confirmed by magnetic resonance imaging. Surgical treatment is necessary to prevent further deterioration after development of a syringomyelia.

Patients need careful periodic monitoring by detailed neurological examination to document any changes in motor or sensory function. As noted above, neurological changes may be due to peripheral entrapments or to development of a syrinx. In either case, treatment should begin at once so that optimal neurological function can be maintained.

Genitourinary System

Mortality and morbidity in the SCI population owing to renal disease has decreased dramatically in the past three decades. This is likely due to refinement of acute care bladder management, the introduction of intermittent catheterization, broad-spectrum antibiotics, and improved long-term surveillance. Late structural and physiological changes in the genitourinary system, however, are not fully understood.

In the general population, changes in the aging genitourinary system include decreased bladder capacity and urethral compliance, increase in residual urine volume, and increase in uninhibited detrusor contractions. Changes in renal function include a decrease in glomerular filtration rates, decreases in renal plasma flow, and changes in diurnal excretory patterns so patients need to urinate at night. Genitourinary problems in the general population also increase with age, and the combination of normal aging changes with a neurogenic bladder will likely complicate bladder management in the aging individual with SCI.

People in both the general aging population and those with SCI are at an increased risk for developing UTIs. The increased incidence of UTIs is associated with age-related changes in the immune system, prostatism, and menopause. Changes in the aging prostate result in increased postvoid bladder residuals and decreased prostatic antibacterial factors. Menopause alters the urinary tract mucosa and increases the potential for bacterial colonization of the vulva. Asymptomatic bacteriuria in the presence of obstructive uropathy or reflux should be treated to prevent pyelonephritis. In the absence of obstruction or reflux, however, use of antibiotics must be weighed against their potential toxic and adverse effects, interactions with other medications, and the narrowed margin between toxic and therapeutic doses in the older people.

Each method of bladder management is associated with certain complications as a person ages. Higher rates of bladder stones, urinary tract infections, and bladder cancer have typically been associated with indwelling catheters. Urethral stricture and epididymitis have been associated with the long-term use of intermittent catheters.

As people with SCI age, changes in fine motor control, visual acuity, and overall endurance may affect their ability to transfer to and from the wheelchair to perform intermittent catheterization and may require modifications in bladder management. Should access to care providers cease, techniques may need to be altered to preserve some independence. Individuals with SCI need to be aware of the problems that may result with specific types of bladder management; modifications in techniques may be necessary.

People with SCI are also at increased risk of developing bladder cancer. Bladder cancer is the fourth most common cancer in men in this country and the fourth most common cause of cancer death. In the general population, the incidence of bladder cancer is 0.018 percent; estimates for those with SCI range between 0.32 and 10 percent. Bladder cancer in people with SCI has been related to bladder irritation owing to recurrent or chronic urinary tract infections, long use of indwelling catheters, urinary tract stones, urinary tract obstruction, cigarette smoking, and certain medications. It has been reported that the overall incidence of bladder cancer in people managed with an indwelling catheter is 9 percent, with those managed for longer than ten years having an incidence of 20 percent (Lanig 1993). People with SCI who develop bladder cancer typically present with hematuria. Since hematuria is also commonly associated with urinary tract infections, bladder stones, and catheter changes, it is not a reliable indicator of bladder cancer. In contrast to the general population, in which transitional cell carcinoma is by far the most frequent histological type, patients with SCI have a higher frequency of histologically mixed squamous and adenocarcinomatous morphology, an aggressive type of tumor that is usually not diagnosed until it is in an advanced stage. Unfortunately, at the time of diagnosis, bladder tumors in those with SCI have often metastasized, highlighting the importance of developing effective early screening methods. Health care professionals need to be more aware of the increased risk of bladder cancer in those with SCI and the importance of early screening.

Changes in Body Composition

SCI predisposes the individual to medical complications and secondary disabilities such as obesity, lipid abnormalities, carbohydrate intolerance, and cardiovascular disease (Bauman 1997). One hypothesis is that these secondary disabilities are the result of adverse changes in body composition. Those with SCI have body composition changes similar to those in aging able-bodied people, including loss of lean tissue mass and increase of fat tissue. After acute

SCI, dramatic reductions in body weight and lean soft tissue occur in regions of the body that are acutely paralyzed. People with chronic SCI have less lean tissue and more fat tissue than able-bodied people. The higher or more complete the spinal cord lesion (the greater the neurological deficit), the greater the decrease in lean body tissue. Conversely, the percentage of body fat rises as the level of neurological deficit increases. In addition, there appears to be a continued loss of lean body tissue and an increase in the percentage of fat tissue with advancing age. In an identical twin study, with one twin in each pair having SCI, it has been reported that a loss of total body and extremity muscle mass was continuous, with greater losses occurring with longer duration of injury.

The loss of lean body tissue is directly reflected in the metabolic rate (Spungen et al. 1993). A strong relation exists between metabolic rate and fat-free mass both in able-bodied people and in those with SCI. The greater the reduction in lean body tissue, the greater the decrease in resting metabolic rate. Not surprisingly, those patients with higher cord lesions generally have lower metabolic rates, presumably owing to greater loss of lean tissue.

Carbohydrate Metabolism

Disorders of oral carbohydrate tolerance are more prevalent in people with SCI than in the able-bodied population (fig. 9.1; Bauman 1997). Most individuals with SCI who have a disorder in glucose tolerance show peripheral resistance of insulin to mediate glucose uptake. The normal response to an elevation of blood glucose in the presence of insulin resistance is increased release of insulin to maintain the blood glucose concentration within the normal range. Even in the absence of any worsening in glucose tolerance, insulin resistance and hyperinsulinemia predispose people to cardiovascular disease. If the body cannot release enough insulin after eating, which may occur with aging, elevations in the serum glucose level will result.

The determinants of insulin action are body composition and level of fitness. Increased body fat is associated with insulin resistance. Studies of body fat topography in able-bodied people have suggested that distribution of body fat may be important in the association of obesity with other metabolic disorders. Fat on the trunk has the most adverse effect on carbohydrate and lipid metabolism. In people with SCI, the usual clinical measures may underestimate adiposity. A reduction in muscle mass will also reduce the effectiveness

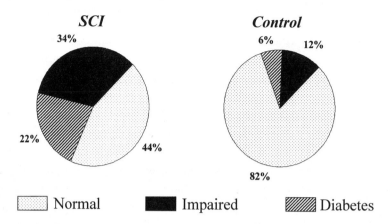

Figure 9.1. Glucose abnormalities in middle-aged persons with spinal cord injury (SCI). *Source:* Adapted with permission from Bauman et al. 1994.

of insulin. Significantly, increasing levels of fitness increase the action of insulin on muscle glucose utilization.

The relation of oral carbohydrate tolerance to level and completeness of lesion has been studied. The subjects with complete tetraplegia had significantly worse carbohydrate tolerance and were more frequently classified with a disorder in carbohydrate tolerance than the other neurological deficit subgroups. Those with complete tetraplegia had higher insulin values after an oral glucose load than groups with lesser neurological deficits. Oral carbohydrate tolerance was similar in men and women, but the plasma insulin levels were higher for men, suggesting they had relative insulin resistance. Glucose abnormalities generally increased with age.

At least three factors are involved in the pathogenesis of type II diabetes mellitus: a genetic predisposition, impaired insulin action, and a defect in pancreatic beta-cell function. The genetic basis of type II diabetes is complex but the tendency to develop diabetes may be increased by environmental causes, such as those present in people with SCI. Insulin resistance is generally present in individuals with a hereditary predisposition to develop impaired glucose tolerance or type II diabetes mellitus. To date, the natural course of impaired glucose tolerance or "mild" diabetes in people with SCI has not been reported. The progression from impaired glucose tolerance to diabetes mellitus depends on many factors, including genetic composition, environment, length of follow-up, and means of assessment.

The average fasting plasma glucose is only mildly elevated in subjects with SCI because peripheral insulin resistance is the major factor responsible for glucose intolerance in this disorder. Subjects with impaired glucose tolerance or diabetes mellitus may have fasting plasma glucose values within the normal range and be without symptoms of any carbohydrate disorder. Thus it is important to perform a formal glucose tolerance test. The currently accepted classifications for diagnosis of the disorders of oral carbohydrate tolerance are those of the Expert Committee on the Diagnosis and Classification of Diabetes Mellitus (Diagnosis and classification of diabetes mellitus 1997). As in the able-bodied population, diabetes mellitus may be associated with unexplained weight loss, blurred vision, and increased frequency of infection as well as the generally recognized symptoms of increased thirst, food intake, and urination. Any individual with SCI should make an effort to reduce the risk of developing diabetes. Obesity, physical inactivity, and a high-fat diet are recognized risk factors for diabetes, and they all can be modified. Combining exercise with diet therapy has been shown to be more effective than either approach alone. Once diabetes mellitus is diagnosed, additional effort must be made to reduce body fat by restricting calories and increasing activity (Position Statement 1997).

Lipid Profile

Elevation in low density lipoprotein (LDL) cholesterol and depression of high density lipoprotein (HDL) cholesterol are two important risk factors for coronary heart disease (CHD). Individuals with SCI are believed to have accelerated and premature CHD. Cardiovascular diseases were reported as the most frequent cause of death among people with SCI of more than thirty years' duration or among those more than sixty years old (Whiteneck et al. 1992). The lipid profile in people with SCI should be determined, and appropriate management should be instituted to reduce risk for CDH.

Approximately 10 percent of the U.S. population has HDL cholesterol values less than 35 mg/dL, which is an independent risk factor for CHD, whereas about 24 to 40 percent of those with SCI have levels below this value. There is an indirect association between abdominal circumference, a surrogate measure of trunk fat, and serum HDL cholesterol levels: the greater the abdominal circumference, the lower the level of serum HDL cholesterol (Maki et al. 1995). Lower levels of serum HDL cholesterol have been found in subjects with chronic tetraplegia than in those with paraplegia. Subjects with motor complete injuries have lower values of serum HDL cholesterol than those with incomplete injuries for either category of level of lesion. While males with SCI have been reported to have lower HDL cholesterol than controls, no significant difference was found for females, who were predominantly premenopausal.

Better cardiopulmonary fitness has been shown to improve serum HDL cholesterol levels in subjects with or without SCI. Lack of activity, independent of lipid values or other risk factors for CHD, may be an independent risk factor for CHD. Patients should be encouraged to reach and maintain the highest level of daily activity compatible with their injury.

The prevalence of elevated levels of serum LDL cholesterol in individuals with SCI is similar to that reported in the able-bodied population. The therapy recommendations of the National Cholesterol Education Program (1993) are based on the level of serum LDL cholesterol in association with the presence or absence of CHD or risk factors for CHD. A complete lipid profile should be performed in all adults who are twenty and older at least once every five years. If values exceed those recommended by the National Cholesterol Education Program, then appropriate therapy should be instituted. A low-fat, low-cholesterol diet and medication may be used to lower elevated serum LDL cholesterol levels.

Anabolic Hormones

A deficiency of "body-building" or anabolic hormones causes adverse changes in soft tissue body composition. The two main anabolic hormones found in the body are testosterone and growth hormone. Although the literature on people with SCI is somewhat controversial, subsets of men with SCI most likely have a relative or absolute deficiency of these hormones (Tsitouras et al. 1995). Serum testosterone levels tend to decrease with age in those with SCI, as has been observed in able-bodied people, and they also decrease with longer duration of injury. Growth hormone and its second messenger, insulinlike growth factor 1 (IGF-1), have been reported to be depressed in individuals with SCI. In a study of people with postpolio syndrome, lower plasma IGF-1 levels were found to be a potent discriminator of those who had decreased capacity to perform activities of daily living, reduced functional independence, and increased pain (Rao et al. 1993). Although it is not possible to determine cause or effect from this investigation, it appears that depressed plasma IGF-1 levels in people with SCI are associated with reductions in muscle mass and strength and hence functional capacity. Therapeutic physiological replacement of endogenous anabolic hormones in the able-bodied population has generally been beneficial. Such clinical interventions in individuals with SCI have been undertaken experimentally in limited trials. In addition to such attempts, anabolic steroids can be used for specific indications in people with SCI. Anabolic steroid administration was associated with improvement in subjective symptoms and objective signs of breathing in subjects with tetraplegia. In addition, case studies have reported that an anabolic agent along with conventional care helped heal refractory pressure ulcers.

Pulmonary Function

Conceptually, the muscles of breathing may be divided into the diaphragm, intercostals/accessory muscles, and the abdominal wall group (Morgan, Silver, and William 1986). These muscles are different from the other skeletal muscles in three aspects: they are both involuntary and voluntary; they overcome resistive and elastic loads rather than inertial loads; and they must contract regularly and indefinitely without prolonged rest. The respiratory muscles work as either prime movers or stabilizers of the chest wall to promote inspiration and exhalation. The inspiratory muscles function in a coordinated effort to enlarge the thoracic cavity, creating a negative intrapleural pressure and inflating the lung. The diaphragm is the primary muscle responsible for inspiration during quiet breathing. Exhalation during quiet breathing is largely passive. The inspiratory action of the diaphragm depends on its configuration and the presence of abdominal resistance. In patients with pulmonary compromise, the diaphragm may flatten, weakening its ability to inspire. The diaphragm is innervated at cervical levels 3, 4, and 5 (fig. 9.2). The accessory muscles include the scalenes, sternocleidomastoids, and trapezius. These muscles contribute minimally to inhalation during tidal breathing and are innervated from the cranial nerve XI to cervical nerve II. The scalenes may play an active role by stabilizing the rib cage during quiet breathing. The intercostals are primarily responsible for forced efforts of inhalation (external intercostals) and exhalation (internal intercostals); these muscles are innervated at thoracic levels 1 through 12 (fig. 9.2) and are recruited to assist with deep inspirations and forceful exhalations. The abdominal wall group

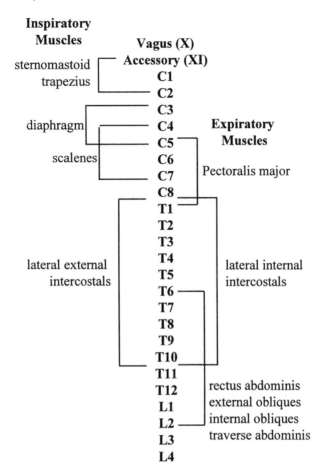

Figure 9.2. Innervation of the muscles of breathing.

consists of the recti, external, and internal obliques and the transverse abdominis. These muscles primarily contract to participate in exhalation at higher levels of ventilation, such as during exercise or stress and during the explosive exhalation of coughing, and they are relatively inactive during quiet breathing. The abdominal wall group is innervated at thoracic level 1 through lumbar level 2. In cases of cervical paralysis, such as seen in those with tetraplegia, the pectoralis major has been shown to participate in exhalation.

Depending on the level and completeness of lesion, SCI has the potential to paralyze the muscles of breathing. Complete cord lesions above thoracic level 5 noticeably reduce pulmonary function, with higher cord lesions causing greater reductions. The inability to adequately inspire or expire owing to paralysis is a form of restrictive lung disease (the lungs are "restricted" from full expansion). Complete cord lesions above cervical level 3 compromise the diaphragm enough to require mechanical ventilation.

Breathlessness is the single most frequently reported respiratory symptom, and it is far more prevalent among patients with tetraplegia than among those with paraplegia. Breathlessness in those with tetraplegia is associated with reduced pulmonary function. The symptoms of coughing, sputum production, and wheezing appear to occur at about the same frequency among subjects with all levels of lesion. A regular program of inspiratory muscle training has been shown to decrease restrictive ventilatory impairment in those with chronic cervical SCI and to reduce respiratory complaints.

In addition to the restrictive impairment that has been well appreciated in those with SCI, people with spinal cord lesions above thoracic level 6 have been shown to have an obstructive or "asthmalike" component to breathing (Spungen et al. 1993). Anecdotally, patients with higher cord lesions often report difficulty breathing when they come into contact with cold air, perfume, or other environmental pollutants. It has been speculated that transection of the spinal cord above the sympathetic outflow to the lung may result in unopposed parasympathetic tone, producing bronchoconstriction. Agents that cause bronchial irritation and bronchoconstriction do so at greatly reduced doses in patients with these higher cord lesions. Bronchodilators (adrenergic or anticholinergic medications) that are routinely used to treat asthma in the able-bodied population , are efficacious in reversing the bronchoconstriction and the enhanced irritability of the airway.

Gastrointestinal Manifestations

SCI has direct and indirect effects on the entire gastrointestinal tract. Autonomic nerve interruption may have direct effects on bowel motility but may also have indirect effects on diet, oral hygiene, bacterial flora, level of activity, and body composition. This discussion will briefly address the major considerations from the oral cavity to the anus.

Because many people with tetraplegia depend on caregivers for daily oral care, they generally have increased plaque, gingivitis, and periodontal disease.

People with SCI may be treated with a wide variety of medications to reduce spasticity of the limbs or the bladder that have generalized anticholinergic side effects, one of which is dry mouth, associated with increased dental caries. Use of a mouthstick in those with tetraplegia applies an unphysiologic force to the teeth that often leads to dental trauma and associated deleterious dental conditions.

Gastroesophageal reflux disease is quite common in people with SCI (specifically higher cord lesions), who spend more of their time either lying down or in the semiupright position (Glickman and Kamm 1996). People with lower cord lesions, who are often constipated, can recruit their abdominal muscles to increase intra-abdominal pressure to assist in defecation, but the maneuver leads to increased relaxation of the lower esophageal sphincter and reflux of gastric contents into the esophagus. Abnormal motility of the esophagus increases the risk of gastric reflux esophagitis by lengthening the exposure of the esophagus to gastric juices. Lifestyle modifications include avoiding foods (chocolate and peppermint), drinks (coffee and alcohol), and activities that increase gastric acidity or irritate the esophagus, as well as elevating the head after meals and not eating before bedtime. Medications may be prescribed to reduce gastric acidity. However, noncompliance is high, resulting in high-grade esophagitis with intractable symptoms and complications such as esophageal stricture and aspiration.

The propulsive contractions of the colon, as well as the act of defecation itself, require sacral parasympathetic and somatic nervous input, which are often altered after upper or lower neuron spinal cord injuries. Neurogenic bowel includes a variety of dysfunctions that include increased bowel transit time, constipation, incontinence, and abnormalities in defecation. The bowel dysfunction should be designated as upper motor neuron or lower motor neuron in etiology. A comprehensive, individualized treatment plan called a bowel program is designed to eliminate incontinence, achieve effective and efficient colonic evacuation, and prevent the secondary complications associated with bowel dysfunction. The bowel program consists of evaluation and intervention with diet, exercise, equipment, oral medications, rectal medications, and schedule of bowel care.

Gallstones are more prevalent in people with SCI. In developed Western countries, the prevalence of cholelithiasis ranges from 5 to 17.5 percent, whereas in those with SCI the prevalence is from 21 to 30 percent. Decreased gallbladder motility has been associated with a higher prevalence of gallstones and sludge. It was hypothesized that contributions to gallbladder motility from the autonomic nervous system may be altered after SCI, which may alter contractibility and result in cholestasis. However, it appears that gallbladder contractility is normal. Thus the etiology of the increased prevalence of disease is unclear, but it may simply be due to an increase in the incidence of conventional risk factors for the disease, such as obesity. Because people with SCI may have interruption of efferent nervous impulses from the region (above thoracic level 7), cholecystitis may present without right upper quadrant pain but with nonspecific gastrointestinal complaints of nausea and vomiting associated with fever. A high index of suspicion is needed to make the diagnosis early, before gangrene of the gallbladder occurs with its high mortality rate. An associated complication of cholelithiasis is gallstone pancreatitis, which may be difficult to diagnose owing to nonspecific abdominal symptoms, loss of visceral sensations, possible associated pulmonary findings (atelectasis and pneumonia), and a low index of suspicion. Elevation of pancreatic enzymes and radiological visualization of the pancreas will support the diagnosis.

Summary

In the United States, there are approximately 200,000 people with SCI. These injuries are categorized by degree of neurological defect. Owing to the introduction of antibiotics and improvements in urological care, people with SCI should have a life expectancy that approaches that of the able-bodied population, but functional and medical problems may occur prematurely.

Immobilization and reduced or absent sensation may cause skin breakdown. The primary way to prevent pressure ulcers is by educating patients in skin inspection, pressure relief, and positioning. Patients' increased energy requirements must be met with adequate protein and caloric intake to promote healing of pressure ulcers. Aging in people with SCI is accompanied by all the musculoskeletal changes that occur in the nondisabled, including decreased muscular strength and function. Osteoarthritis may occur earlier in people with SCI because they need to use their upper extremities for mobility, locomotion, and exercise. Disuse osteoporosis results in long bones that are prone to fracture with minor trauma. Efforts should be made to maintain adequate vitamin D and calcium intake. Entrapment neuropathies are prevalent in the wrist owing to repetitive motions of the wrist and hand, as well as frequent trauma to the region. A late neurological deterioration may be due to posttraumatic syringomyelia.

Great strides in gentiourinary care have increased the longevity of those with paralysis. Bladder management techniques must be appropriate if the individual is to maintain health and preserve function and independence. Individuals with SCI are at an increased risk of developing urinary tract infections, urinary tract stones, and bladder cancer. The bladder cancer that develops in those with SCI is more aggressive and lethal than that usually diagnosed in the able-bodied population.

As a consequence of relative inactivity and body composition changes, people with SCI are predisposed to metabolic abnormalities in carbohydrate and lipid metabolism. A deficiency of endogenous anabolic hormones—growth hormone and testosterone—may worsen these changes. Physiological replacement with testosterone may be considered. Anabolic steroid hormones may have specific indications for therapy for a circumscribed period. There is a markedly increased prevalence of glucose intolerance and diabetes mellitus. The primary lipid abnormality is a depressed HDL cholesterol concentration. These metabolic complications may be addressed with appropriate diet, physical activity, and medications.

SCI may cause respiratory muscle paralysis. The higher and more complete the lesion, the greater the compromise to breathing. The inability to expand the lungs is referred to as restrictive lung disease. Lesions above cervical level 4 may impair diaphram function enough to require mechanical ventilation. Breathlessness is the most common symptom of individuals with SCI, and those with tetraplegia have significantly more symptoms than those with paraplegia. Obstructive lung disease or an "asthmalike" condition has been described in those with paralysis above thoracic level 6. Environmental irritants may more easily precipitate bronchospasm in such individuals. Bronchodilators will provide symptomatic relief.

SCI causes gastrointestinal morbidity. Gingivitis and periodontal disease are frequent. Gastroesophageal reflux disease is primarily due to supine posture, but increased abdominal pressure associated with difficult stool evacuation may contribute. Bowel care programs should be individualized to maximize fecal continence and independence. The increased prevalence of acute and chronic gallbladder disease should be recognized.

REFERENCES

American Spinal Injury Association/International Medical Society of Paraplegia (ASIA/IMSOP). 1996. *International standards for neurological and functional classification of SCI.* (Revised 1996.) Chicago: ASIA.

Bauman, W. A. 1997. Carbohydrate and lipid metabolism in individuals after spinal cord injury. *Topics in Spinal Cord Injury Rehabilitation* 2:1–22.

Bauman, W. A., Garland, D., and Schwartz, E. 1997. Calcium metabolism and osteoporosis in individuals after spinal cord injury. *Topics in Spinal Cord Injury Rehabilitation* 2:84–95.

Bauman, W. A., Zhong, Y. G., and Schwartz, E. 1995. Vitamin D deficiency in veterans with chronic SCI. *Metabolism* 44:1612–16.

Bauman, W. A., et al. 1994. *Metabolism* 43:749–56.

Consortium for Spinal Cord Medicine. 2000. Pressure ulcer prevention and treatment following spinal cord injury: A clinical practice guideline for health-care professionals. Paralyzed Veterans of America.

Demling, R. H., and DeSanti, L. 1998. Closure of the "non-healing wound" corresponds with correction of weight loss using the anabolic agent oxandrolone. *Ostomy/Wound Management* 44:58–68.

Glickman, S., and Kamm, M. A. 1996. Bowel dysfunction in spinal cord injured patients. *Lancet* 347:1651–53.

Lanig, I. S. 1993. The genitourinary system. In *Aging with SCI*, ed. G. Whiteneck, S. W. Charlifue, K. A. Gerhart, et al., 105-15. New York: Demos.

Maki, K. C., Briones, E. R., Langbein, W. E., Inman-Felton, A., Nemchausky, B. M., and Burton, J. 1995. Associations between serum lipids and indicators of adiposity in men with spinal cord injury. *Paraplegia* 33 (2): 102–9.

Morgan, M. D. L., Silver, J. R., and William, S. J. 1986. The respiratory system of the spinal cord patient. In *Management of spinal cord injury*, ed. R. F. Bloch and M. Basbaum, 78-116. Baltimore: Williams and Wilkins.

Nash, M. S., and Fletcher, M. 1993. The immune system. In *Aging with SCI*, ed. G. Whiteneck, S. W. Charlifue , K. A. Gerhart, et al., 159-81. New York: Demos.

National Cholesterol Education Program. 1993. Summary of the second report of the National Cholesterol Education Program (NCEP) Expert Panel on Detection, Evaluation, and Treatment of High Blood Cholesterol in Adults (Adult Treatment Panel II). *JAMA* 269:3015–23.

Pentland, W. E., and Twomey, L. 1994. Upper limb function in persons with long term paraplegia and implications for independence: Part II. *Paraplegia* 32:219–24.

Position statement: Nutritional recommendations and principles for individuals with diabetes mellitus. 1997. *Diabetes Care* 14:20–27.

Report of the Expert Committee on the Diagnosis and Classification of Diabetes Mellitus. 1997. *Diabetes Care* 20:1183–97.

Rao, U., Shetty, K. R., Mattson, D. E., Rudman, I. W., and Rudman, D. 1993. Prevalence of low plasma IGF-I in poliomyelitis survivors. *Journal of American Geriatric Society* 41:697–702.

Spungen, A. M., Bauman, W. A., Wang, J., and Peirson, R. N., Jr. 1993. The relationship between total body potassium and resting energy expenditure in individuals with paraplegia. *Archives of Physical Medicine and Rehabilitation* 74:965-68.

Spungen, A. M., Dicpinigaitis, P. V., Almenoff, P. L., and Bauman, W. A. 1993. Pulmonary obstruction in individuals with cervical spinal cord lesions unmasked by bronchodilators. *Paraplegia* 31:404–7.

Stewart, A. F., Adler, M., Byers, C. M., Segre, G. V., and Broadus, A. E. 1982. Calcium homeostasis in immobilization: An example of resorptive hypercalciuria. *New England Journal of Medicine* 306 (19): 113

Tsitouras, P. D., Zhong, Y. G., Spungen, A. M., and Bauman, W. A. 1995. Serum testosterone and growth hormone/insulin-like growth factor-I in adults with spinal cord injury. *Hormone Metabolic Research* 27:287–92.

Waters, R. L., and Sie, I. H. 2001. Upper extremity changes with SCI contrasted to common aging in the musculoskeletal system. *Topics in Spinal Cord Rehabilitation* 6:61–68.

Waters, R. L., Sie, I. H., and Adkins, R. H. 2001. The musculoskeletal system. *Topics in Spinal Cord Rehabilitation* 6:vii–viii.

Whiteneck, G. G., Charlifue, S. W., Frankel, H. L., Fraser, M. H., Gardner, B. P., Gerhart, K. A., Krishnan, K. R., Menter, R. R., Nuseibeh, I., Short, D. J., and Silver, J. R. 1992. Mortality, morbidity, and psychosocial outcomes of persons spinal cord injured more than 20 years ago. *Paraplegia* 30:617–30.

10

Aging with Poliomyelitis

Jacquelin Perry, M.D., D.Sc. (Hon.)

Poliomyelitis is an ancient, worldwide paralyzing disease caused by poliovirus invasion of the nervous system during periodic epidemics. The functional outcome, while ranging from complete healing to multiple levels of residual paralysis, was assumed to be a stable situation. However, time has revealed significant late effects of polio that can lead to functional instability.

Initial Disability (Acute Poliomyelitis)

Initially, the disease was called infantile paralysis because the virus mainly attacked children younger than five years (Edwards, Clark, and Drake 1958). By the 1934 epidemic, improved sanitation had reduced people's immunity sufficiently that more adults were affected, leading to a greater incidence of extensive paralysis and less complete recovery.

The acute clinical picture typically began with severe flulike symptoms accompanied by pain, back and neck stiffness, and varying extent of paralysis. Based on the use of manual muscle testing to detect paralysis, approximately one-third of the patients were diagnosed as nonparalytic (Spencer 1954). Of the paralytic patients, 70 percent were classified as spinal; their paralysis involved the muscles of the neck, chest, trunk, and limbs. Involvement of one or more of the cranial nerves, which arise at the base of the brain, was called bulbar polio (10 percent). Combined involvement was classed as bulbospinal (20 percent) (Spencer 1954).

Both the severity and the extent of the paralysis varied markedly among individuals, though the initial paresis was usually profound. In a group of 142 patients, 74 percent of the lower limbs had severe involvement of most muscles, while just 44 percent of the upper limbs had even one-fourth of their muscles involved (Sharrard 1955). Full body impairment occurred in 4 percent of the patients (Edwards, Clark, and Drake 1958). The potential for recovery varied individually but grossly followed two courses. About 10 percent of the patients regained normal function within two to four weeks (Edwards, Clark, and Drake 1958). The gains in strength were significantly slower by the third month and became less each month, with patients attaining 93 percent recovery in one year. During the slow recovery period, the average lower-extremity muscle gain was two grades, while the upper-extremity muscles did slightly better, averaging a 2.5 grade gain.

Bulbar polio was of two types. Paresis of the upper nerves (I–VII) caused specific loss of eye or face muscle function. However, impairment of the lower nerves (VIII–XII), which controlled the tongue and swallowing, was ominous for survival because of their importance in saliva, food, and airway management (Edwards, Clark, and Drake 1958). Also, viral invasion of this area could alter consciousness or anxiety level, leading to the diagnosis of polioencephalitis (Spencer 1954). Survival of a small percentage of patients with spinal lesions also was threatened by paralysis of the respiratory muscles, particularly the diaphragm. Fatality averaged 7 percent.

Acute Pathology

The underlying neuropathology was identified by experimentally induced polio in monkeys (Bodian 1949). Detailed analysis showed that the virus primarily invaded two areas: the spinal cord and the brain stem. Rarely were any pathological changes found in the cerebral or cerebellar cortex except for an occasional mild lesion in the motor cortex (Bodian 1949).

In the spinal cord the viral invasion concentrated on the anterior horn area, which contained the motor nerve cells to the skeletal muscles. Involvement of the adjacent areas was spotty and rarely symptomatic. The virus invaded about 95 percent of the motor cells. In areas of severe infection, motor cell death and absorption were rapid, occurring within the first two to three days, followed by muscle atrophy about two weeks later. Cells that were injured but not destroyed regained normal morphology within a month. The incidence of spinal motor cell destruction by the poliovirus ranged from 12 percent to 91 percent, with an average of 47 percent (Bodian 1985). Thus, while some patients experienced a minor deficit, most were left with a significant neurological loss. Superimposed on this deficit was considerable disuse muscle atrophy resulting from the prolonged hospitalization used to protect the recovering neuromuscular system from strain.

In the patients with bulboencephalitis, viral invasion of the brain stem in the area of the reticular formation and adjacent nuclei was the source of their restlessness, drowsiness, or coma (Bodian 1949). Electrical stimulation studies showed that the reticular system activated the entire brain, with particular responsibility for normal wakefulness (Guyton 1971). The normal stimulation of the reticular activation system is from signals generated by the joints and muscles, skin, eyes, ears, and viscera, with pain and proprioception being the most potent.

Function was regained by three mechanisms: muscle hypertrophy, axon sprouting, and coping. Accelerated exercise and resumption of function substituted hypertrophy for disuse atrophy.

Axon sprouting significantly enlarged the neural pool. This neurological response was overlooked during the acute polio era because the original research related to peripheral nerve injuries, and it occurred late in the polio era (Weiss and Edds 1946). The investigators found that partial nerve injuries stimulated increased sprouting of the remaining axons to reinnervate the muscle fibers that had lost their primary nerve supply. A fourfold increase in the population of functioning muscle fibers was identified (fig. 10.1A, B). In poliomyelitis this probably is source of the slow gains in muscle strength that followed the initial period of cell healing.

Coping with the permanent polio residuals proved very effective. Using their normal mental alertness, peripheral proprioception, and cerebral motor control, the recovering polio patients devised ways of regaining lost function through substitutive action. By adaptive posturing, ligament tension replaced inactive musculature for stance stability, and swing motion was gleaned from remote muscle action such as a twist of the trunk to advance the leg in walking or the arm for reach. All but the most severely impaired patients discarded their orthoses during their teen years. Often this progress was assisted by reconstructive orthopedic surgery to stabilize joints or redistribute muscle control. Even patients with severe permanent paralysis who continued to depend on orthoses, walking aids, wheelchairs, or personal assistance found ways to hold jobs and to prove they were as able as their colleagues. They successfully blended into all facets of society as normal, contributing persons. An epidemi-

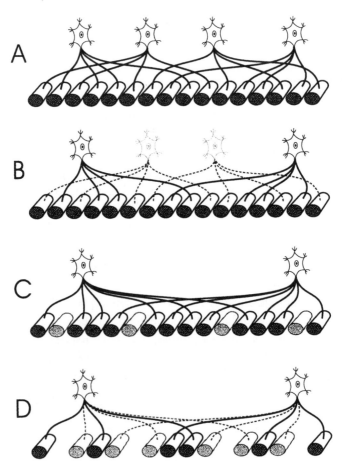

Figure 10.1. Motor unit innervation patterns. A, Normal, four anterior horn cells with each innervating four muscle fibers. B, Acute poliovirus destruction of two anterior horn cells (faint) with loss of their axon sprouts (dashed). C, Remaining motor cells send out additional axon sprouts to reinnervate most of the orphaned muscle fibers. D, Late loss of axon sprouts and muscle fibers from chronic overuse. Gray shading indicates lost fibers.

ological study of 551 people with confirmed polio showed that 32 percent recovered with no permanent residuals. Among the 78 percent with residual paresis, one-third used an ambulatory aid, 4 percent required a wheelchair, and 1 percent used a respirator (Ramlowet al. 1992). Within the paretic group, 35 percent participated in high school sports, and most felt they equaled their peers. Most also had some education beyond high school. Only 1 percent were unable to work.

Nationwide introduction of the Salk vaccine in 1955 abruptly terminated the polio epidemics in the United States and gradually reduced the incidence of polio worldwide. Introduction of the Sabin oral vaccine removed the need for needle injection, making the preventive program much more acceptable. Also, as an attenuated live vaccine, its immunization included the contacts of the inoculated person (herd vaccination). Unfortunately, an occasional highly susceptible person developed a full case of polio. In the United States this averaged ten cases a year. Return to the killed-virus Salk vaccination has eliminated this problem. Since 1998 there have been no new polio cases in the United States.

Late Effects of Aging (Postpolio Syndrome)

After years of stable function, an increasing number of polio survivors noted new disabling symptoms. While cases of late loss of strength had been reported in the world literature since 1875, they were too isolated to arouse concern (Perry, Barnes, and Gronley 1988). Nationwide population growth and the increasing incidence of major epidemics between 1935 and 1954, however, created a large reservoir of polio survivors (Edwards, Clark, and Drake 1958). In the late 1970s, signs of a significant problem began to emerge. Lacking an organized base of knowledge, the medical profession was ill equipped to respond.

Several surveys explored the nature of the postpolio problem. In southern California, new patients began arriving at a nearly dormant polio orthopedic clinic with complaints of more than broken braces. Of the 193 patients seen in 1979-84, 23 percent complained of increased muscle weakness, and 40 percent were experiencing joint pain. Their average age was forty-two years (eighteen to seventy-five) and the average postpolio interval was twenty-five years (sixteen to sixty-seven). Ninety percent were ambulatory, of whom 42 percent used no aid. Residual paresis was 65 percent lower extremity, 28 percent upper extremity, and 7 percent spine (Perry and Fleming 1985). A 1983 questionnaire survey of polio survivors in the New York City area presented a more severely involved and older group (Halstead and Rossi 1985). Only 47 percent could walk, and 26 percent required a ventilator. Their average age was fifty-three years, with a thirty-four-year postpolio interval. Their complaints were increased muscle weakness (87 percent), fatigue (87 percent), breathing difficulty (58 percent), and muscle and joint pain (79 percent). Walking and climbing stairs (70 percent), transfers (39 percent), and dressing (27 percent) were more difficult. Most of these respondents were survivors of the 1949 polio epidemic.

Two population-based surveys of polio survivors avoided the bias of voluntary participation. Of the 248 living polio survivors in Olmsted County, Minnesota, 21 percent admitted to new symptoms (Windebank, Litchy, and Daube 1995). A more detailed study of 50 survivors living close to Rochester, Minnesota, identified 64 percent with various combinations of weakness, fatigue, and pain. Their average age was fifty years and their postpolio interval thirty-seven years. All were ambulatory, and 10 percent required additional equipment. In Allegheny County, Pennsylvania, 551 polio survivors were identified, of whom 78 percent had at least one new symptom and 42 percent had decreased capacity in at least one activity of daily living (Ramlow et al. 1992). The diagnosis of the postpolio syndrome was restricted to the 28 percent who suffered both increased muscle weakness and muscle pain (or new difficulty in swallowing). The "nonparalytic" survivors reported the same complaints but with half the frequency. In all four studies there were more women than men, yet in the California polio public health statistics the incidence of acute polio was higher in males. The apparent greater susceptibility of women to late muscle loss may relate to the fact that men naturally have a greater percentage of muscle and women store proportionally more fat. The conclusion from these four reports, representing widely dispersed geographic samples, is that new muscle weakness is not an uncommon late development in polio survivors, and the incidence appeared to increase with the severity of the polio residual. The cause, however, was not apparent.

Performance Qualities

The great variation in the severity of acute polio combined with differing lifestyles means that some survivors developed new symptoms while others did not. This created two postpolio populations: the symptomatic and the asymptomatic. Measurements of knee extension strength of fifty postpolio subjects (two-thirds symptomatic) with grades 4 to 5 by manual muscle testing showed significant differences between the symptomatic and asymptomatic polio survivors when compared with a nonpolio control group (Agre and Rodriguez 1990). The strength of the asymptomatic subjects averaged 80 percent of the nonpolio controls, while the symptomatic subjects had only 60 percent strength. The finding that even the asymptomatic polio survivors had some identifiable weakness is compatible with Bodian's description of the acute pathology (95 percent involvement and a residual loss of at least 10 percent). This suggests susceptibility to developing symptoms in time.

These two groups of polio survivors also differed in their acute polio characteristics. The asymptomatic survivors were younger at onset (five versus eight years). The need for hospitalization was much less (one month versus five months), and the time to maximum recovery was shorter (five versus eight years).

A second diagnostic finding was that manual muscle testing did not differentiate the symptomatic from the asymptomatic polio survivors. This is explained by a study of manual muscle testing capability that showed that the push force of female examiners (physicians and therapists) averaged only 60 percent of normal female knee extension strength. The male examiners had similar limited success when testing men (Mulroy et al. 1997). When testing the opposite sex, the female examiners sensed only 40 percent of the available strength, while the male examiners could match the strength of the female subjects. Only when the polio survivors were weaker than these thresholds did the examiner identify a functional limitation.

Rate of Strength Decline

Attempts to measure the rate of functional loss have been elusive. Most studies have focused on the knee extensors (quadriceps) because subject stabilization is easiest and the stationary dynomometer systems are reliable. Test intervals of one year or less have failed to identify a change. A longitudinal study of thirty polio survivors for quadriceps strength at four and eight years was able to show a change at both testing sessions (Grimby et al. 1998). The subjects who had noted a loss of strength had average declines of 14 percent and 19 percent, while the polio survivors who perceived no weakness showed a 7 percent decrease after eight years. For the whole postpolio group, quadriceps strength averaged 61 percent. By manual muscle testing this would be grade 5 and would be missed on clinical examination. The age-matched controls averaged a 4 percent decline in knee extensor strength. The complaints of the 70 percent of the polio survivors who were symptomatic were fatigue (65 percent), weakness (50 percent), and muscle pain (45 percent). Walking and climbing stairs were more difficult.

Hand dynomometer strength testing of fifteen bilateral muscle groups in the upper (nine) and lower extremities (six) of 120 polio survivors showed significant strength decline at each of two testing sessions separated by three to five months (Klein et al. 2000). In the upper extremities all muscle groups displayed some degree of strength loss, averaging 5 percent per test interval. The lower extremities showed two patterns of response. All of the flexor muscle groups registered some strength loss, averaging 8 percent per test. In contrast, the extensor muscle groups did not display a loss, a finding consistent with the other short-duration studies. Perusal of the data revealed no functional or anatomical pattern to the strength changes. While two-thirds of both the upper and the lower limbs were symptomatic, only 35 percent of the polio survivors were aware of any residual upper-extremity weakness from their acute polio, while 83 percent reported incomplete recovery in their lower extremities.

The rapid rate of muscle weakening displayed in this study may be a wake-up call, or it could relate to the reported incidence of pain during testing (37 percent for the upper extremities) or the duration of the procedure (thirty maximum efforts per subject). Not infrequently, patients in the clinic decline subsequent muscle testing on a follow-up visit because it took them weeks to recover from the first session. Carryover symptoms also could lessen the response at the next testing session. There are two possible explanations for the absence of an extensor muscle response. First is the inability to adequately challenge the subject's muscle strength because it exceeded the examiner's push force (as discussed earlier). Second, the eccentric nature of weight-bearing muscle function may expose the fibers to less strain. This latter interpretation is challenged by EMG gait studies showing that polio survivors exert more intense and more prolonged extensor muscle action during walking than normal subjects (Perry, Barnes, and Gronley 1988).

Respiratory Insufficiency

Adults normally experience a slow decline in breathing capacity, but for polio survivors the decline occurs twice as fast (1.8 percent versus 1 percent per year) (Bach and Alba 2001). This has often led to a need for mechanical respiratory assistance an average of twenty-nine years after acute polio. At that time, their mean age was forty-two years. All but two of the seventy-one survivors studied had initially required at least temporary ventilator aid. The effect of increasing respiratory muscle weakness had been aggravated by several comorbidities:

lung disease, obesity, kyphoscoliosis, and cough muscle failure that allowed chronic mucus plugs to accumulate, leading to secondary pneumonia.

Sleep disorder breathing (sleep apnea), which occurs in about 32 percent of nonpolio adults, is more frequent in polio survivors owing to bulbar polio residuals of swallowing muscle weakness and damage to the respiratory center (Bach and Alba 2001). Cardiac failure can result. The critical therapeutic approach is ventilator assistance rather than simple oxygen therapy, since it is essential to correct carbon dioxide retention. Polio survivors anticipating surgery should have a pulmonary function test. Persons with a vital capacity less than 65 percent of normal may be susceptible to anesthetic complications. Opiates and muscle relaxants should be avoided.

Dysphagia

Impaired swallowing was found in 23 percent of 539 subjects surveyed by questionnaire (Halstead and Rossi 1985). A detailed study of twenty polio survivors with current swallowing difficulties revealed that half of them had had acute impairment and half of this group had never fully recovered (Silbergleit, Waring, and Sullivan 1991). Speech was altered in only two. All reported more noticeable difficulty with speech, chewing, and swallowing when fatigued. Videofluoroscopy was used to identify the subjects' swallowing dysfunction and to evaluate the effectiveness of the compensatory strategies recommended. This also was the best diagnostic tool. In response to a follow-up questionnaire one year later, fourteen people reported that they regularly used the recommended strategies and had good results. The major techniques were turning the head, making a dry swallow after each bite, alternating thin liquids with solids, and tilting the head down.

Depression

A comparison of 173 polio survivors and 121 age-matched controls demonstrated that the incidence of depression in polio survivors was not greater than the normal range (Kemp, Adams, and Campbell 1997). When the analysis focused on significant depressive signs, however, such signs were found more frequently in the polio survivors (28 percent) than normal, and the incidence was greater in the symptomatic polio survivors. Berlly, Strausser, and Hall (1991) identified a similar pattern.

Life Satisfaction

Satisfaction with one's life, health, and economic status was lower for polio survivors than for the control subjects, yet more than 50 percent scored above the norm. Acceptance of disability and family support were strong determinants of polio survivors' satisfaction level (Kemp, Adams, and Campbell 1997).

Postpolio Syndrome Pathology

When the surveys reported that polio survivors had begun experiencing loss of function after years of stability, there were no clues to the cause of their new muscle weakness and fatigue. Recent research has significantly clarified the mechanisms of these disabilities. Atrophy of individual muscle fibers is the commonly assumed cause of the new muscle weakness. Counteracting this are numerous muscle biopsy studies showing hypertrophy of the polio muscle fibers (Spector et al. 1996; Grimby et al. 1998). Average postpolio muscle fiber size was 1.7 times larger than in the controls (Grimby et al. 1998). Gross muscle loss, however, with secondary fatty replacement has been demonstrated by magnetic resonance image (MRI) cross sections (fig. 10.2) (Tollback et al. 1996). Hence clinical atrophy is a sign of total muscle loss, not just fiber shrinkage. The loss of muscle mass was conspicuous in many patients with grade 3+ quadriceps.

There is increasing support for the assumption that the new muscle weakness is the result of excessive motor unit enlargement and secondary overuse failure of the axon sprouts (fig. 10.1C, D). Motor unit enlargement is demonstrated by high-amplitude electromyography (EMG) waveforms. Macro EMG has shown that amplitude averages are six to eleven times that for the controls (Grimby et al. 1998), notably greater than the fourfold increase in motor unit size identified in the early peripheral nerve studies (Weiss and Edds 1946). This is interpreted as evidence that the motor nerve cells activate correspondingly more muscle fibers through axon sprouting. A threshold of a twentyfold enlargement was identified as creating a demand that exceeded the available capillary blood supply.

The pattern of strength change secondary to overuse of a partially denervated muscle and its neuronal basis have been demonstrated by serially tabulating the percentage of collateral sprouting at the motor end plates of the

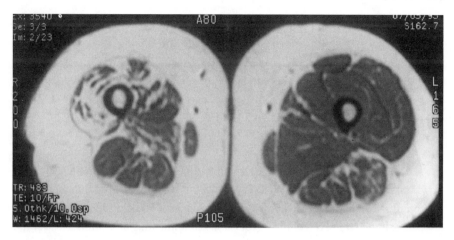

Figure 10.2. Late quadriceps muscle quality in a patient with postpolio syndrome, displayed by magnetic resonance image (MRI) transverse section. Dark area is muscle, light area is fat. Left: Muscle loss and gross fatty replacement are profound in the lateral head of the quadriceps and significant through the rest of the muscle. Clinical grade was 3+. The hamstrings (posterior mass) appear well preserved. Right: Quadriceps muscle area appears normal, clinical grade 5. Hamstrings display moderate loss and fatty replacement, clinical grade 4. Note that the thick subcutaneous fat layer bilaterally obscures the relative thigh atrophy.

rat soleus muscle (Patcher and Eberstein 1995). The immediate response to division of one of the nerve roots supplying the soleus was a reduction in the number of contacts on the motor end plate. At subsequent weeks there was a progressive increase and then later loss in the number of collateral sprouts. Muscle fiber area and strength followed the magnitude of collateral sprouting. The corresponding clinical phases would be the acute polio loss, convalescent recovery of function, and overuse loss of the postpolio syndrome.

The presence of overuse symptoms in muscles presumed to have never been affected by polio is supported by clinical EMG evidence of the typical chronic partial denervation signs of prior polio. This is further confirmation that acute polio was a total body disease.

While all the surveys of the late effects of polio identify fatigue as a leading complaint, it also is a frequent problem for people who have not had polio. "Tiredness" or "lack of energy to do things" and "inability to concentrate" are descriptions of fatigue given by both polio survivors and a control group (Berlly, Strauser, and Hall 1991). The added complaints of "increased physical weakness" and "mild exercise worsening their fatigue" identified by the polio survivors contrasted sharply with the reports of the control group, who often get relief with exercise.

An investigation into the mechanics of fatigue generation and recovery showed that the higher levels of resistance were less tolerated by the symptomatic polio survivors than by age-matched nonpolio subjects (Sunnerhagen et al. 2000). Beyond the fifth step (50 percent maximal voluntary contraction [MVC]) of ten repetitions each, the polio survivors failed to generate a force greater than their 50 percent maximum even though the continuing rise in EMG indicated that they were trying to meet the higher demands. The controls reached the 70 percent MVC level but not the goal of 80 percent maximum. Throughout the exercise, the rise in EMG of the postpolio subjects was at half the rate of the control group's signal, indicating activation of fewer motor units (Sunnerhagen et al. 2000). The investigators interpreted this as a reduction in central drive, but it more likely reflected the relative efficiency of the enlarged motor units documented by macro EMG.

The fatigue rate was not significantly different between the two groups, though maximum postpolio muscle strength was only 67 percent of the control group's. But recovery from the fatigue by the polio survivors was significantly delayed (Sunnerhagen et al. 2000). A second study that compared postpolio groups showed that the symptomatic polio survivors had a major delay in recovering from fatigue, whereas the asymptomatic survivors did not differ significantly from the control subjects (Agre and Rodriguez 1990).

Fatigue also is related to polio muscle energetics. By magnetic resonance spectroscopy, the rate of fuel depletion (loss of phosphocreatine) in the polio muscles was found to be twice that of the control group during an aerobic exercise sequence (Sivakumar et al. 1995). Muscle biopsy analysis identified loss of the oxidative enzyme. These findings indicate that a polio-impaired muscle is partially obligated to use the much less efficient anaerobic process (glycolysis) to generate muscle force. The difference in efficiency between the oxygen-free and oxygenated energizing systems is two versus thirty-two molecules of energy from each molecule of glucose metabolized. Perceived fatigue also was twice as great in the polio survivors. If one applies such muscle inefficiency to the excessive intensity and duration of hip, knee, and calf muscle action during walking documented by gait EMG (Perry, Barnes, and Gronley 1988), the source of daily fatigue is evident. Chronic overuse mechanics of the postpolio syndrome have reduced the effectiveness of the muscles and increased the stress on the controlling neurons. These findings confirm that postpolio fatigue is a physical phenomenon.

"Brain fatigue" is another postpolio complaint. The polio survivors describe it as difficulty with finding words, thinking clearly, and cognition, as well as lapses in attention and memory. Bruno attributes this to damage of the reticular activity system in the brain stem (Bruno et al. 1994). In an MRI study of twenty-two polio survivors, 36 percent had punctuate areas of hyperintense signal, an incidence significantly greater than chance. These subjects, however, represent only half of the group reporting fatigue by questionnaire. An alternative source of "brain fatigue" could be less input to the reticular activating system from the physical fatigue of overused muscles and associated joint pain.

Treatment

Exercise was a conspicuous part of the patients' initial rehabilitation. Also, middle-aged persons "naturally" have less strength owing to changes in lifestyle. Hence strengthening exercise has been a common choice for the new postpolio weakness. Several polio survivors attending clinic had instituted their own exercise program but sought medical help because they felt worse rather than better.

Countering this approach is a vague history that overexercise in acute polio led to strength loss. Also, the symptoms of the postpolio syndrome have developed while these polio survivors still were very active in midlife careers. In response to these latter arguments, a program of lifestyle modification to reduce stress has been advocated. Substitution of orthoses and other aids also is commonly prescribed to replace lost muscle strength or to protect painful joints. Each approach has its own criteria.

The mechanics of living involve considerable muscular effort each day. The arms lift, push, and pull objects of multiple sizes and weight. The legs move the body from one location to another as well as providing support for the arms' function.

Beyond the normal requirements of living, most polio survivors have the added challenge of some degree of residual paresis that they have masked by working harder. Even with obvious residual disability, polio survivors found ways to prove they were as capable as their nonparalytic colleagues. Unfortunately, their aggressive, physically demanding coping strategy has overtaxed their enlarged motor units and led to the postpolio syndrome.

Now, to preserve their remaining function, the symptomatic polio survivors must learn a new coping system (lifestyle modification). The areas to be emphasized are determined from the history of their acute involvement (rate and extent of recovery), their current symptoms, present muscle strength profile, and any comorbidities.

The goal is to avoid overuse by establishing a protective balance between ability (current strength) and demand (lifestyle). Ability is measured by manual testing of the major muscles. When a grade 5 muscle is symptomatic, a stationary dynamometry is scheduled. It is essential to test more than the area of complaint because polio survivors so cleverly substitute one muscle group for another. For the upper extremities, the critical muscle functions are shoulder elevation, external rotation and depression, elbow flexion and extension, and hand grip. For the lower extremities, the critical muscle functions are hip extension and abduction, knee extension, ankle dorsiflexion, and plantar flexion.

Demand is documented by reviewing the person's workday, household, self-care, and recreational activities, seeking those that can be modified or eliminated to reduce the strain while preserving productive living (Young 1991).

In the home, a basic need is to transfer heavy household chores to others (family support is a great asset). Organize tasks to reduce the number of errands needed; stop volunteering for those many "little" tasks; build two or three rest periods into the day. Even ten- or twenty-minute breaks are helpful. Changing tasks can be one form of rest (Young 1991).

At work, the need is to lessen the demands of a typical eight-hour workday. Jobs that were easily managed twenty-five years ago now are threatened by pain and fatigue (McNeal, Somerville, and Wilson 1999). Reduction of this stress begins with the polio survivor's identifying the specific activities that cause pain or fatigue, because the solutions also are specific. Rehabilitation occupational therapists are particularly skilled in this analysis. A survey of fifty polio survivors grouped the solutions into five categories. Buying better fitting furniture or more helpful equipment was the most frequent answer. Generally the cost was less than $500, and 60 percent was provided by the employer. Job modification most often consisted of having their coworkers help with the heavy tasks. Reduced or flexible schedules were infrequent measures. The principal architectural adaptation was assigning a parking place close to the entrance. The workers adopted energy conservation and pacing by task organization.

While many of these solutions necessitated cooperation by employers, supervisors, and coworkers, a survey of these people showed that the percentage with a negative reaction was less than the percentage who were unaware of the need to accommodate a worker's physical limitations (18 percent and 27 percent for employers). Unawareness might have been sustained because 42 percent of the polio survivors were reluctant to ask for any accommodation. The positive finding was that 76 percent of them found their ability to continue working was significantly improved by the accommodations provided.

The most effective means of reducing postpolio syndrome work strain is retirement. The daily eight hours of obligatory activity are avoided, but there also is significant reduction in income. Accepting this restriction is a strong indicator that the polio survivor no longer can meet the physical demands of work. This is a decision that should be supported. Detailed medical documentation will be needed.

Losing weight can dramatically reduce symptoms. It often is claimed that exercise must accompany dieting, but many patients have demonstrated that this is not true. The key factor is to reduce the volume of food eaten. Portions should be no larger than the back of one's hand. Replacing fats and sweets with vegetables and some fruit adds energy by improving health.

If symptomatic polio survivors are to accept such a change in lifestyle, they must become knowledgeable about the pathology of the postpolio syndrome and the consequences of not changing. Hence education is the first step in the lifestyle modification program. Denial often is the immediate reaction; it has been their habit for forty years. Time to reflect on the consequences in the interval before the next one or two clinic visits usually generates cooperation.

A two-year follow-up study of seventy-seven survivors with postpolio syndrome measured program effectiveness by the change in muscle strength (Peach and Olejnik 1991). Muscle strength was graded on a 0-1 numerical scale. Those who fully complied with the recommended program had an average improvement in muscle strength of +0.6 percent annually. Those who only partially complied had some improvement in symptoms, but muscle strength declined 1.3 percent annually. Those who failed to comply had either no improvement or worsening of their symptoms and a 2 percent annual decline in muscle strength.

An unresolved issue is whether strengthening exercise is therapeutic or injurious for symptomatic polio survivors. Several exercise programs have been tested. The purpose of each was to demonstrate that a carefully designed exercise protocol could increase muscle strength without causing harm. An early program of strengthening exercise without concern for fatigue caused further weakening and loss of function in muscles identified as postpolio by EMG, while muscles with simple disuse weakness gained (Feldman and Soskolne 1987). A change to a nonfatiguing, low-intensity, high-repetition exercise protocol for three to six months was more effective. Among thirty-one muscles in six patients, half improved in strength. The others showed no change (Feldman and Soskolne 1987).

At the other end of the exercise spectrum was a short-term, high-resistance quadriceps and elbow extensor strengthening program (Spector et al. 1996). Fatigue was monitored and eccentric effort minimized. Selected for the study were six polio survivors able to do heavy resistance exercise. Their average strength was 61 percent normal. Five of the six averaged a 60 percent gain in quadriceps strength, of which at least 20 percent was present six months later. No changes in function were identified (Spector et al. 1996). The initial elbow extensor response was similar but with less persistence. Susceptibility to overuse was implied by the person who made no gain and was confirmed by the 20 percent decline noted at the six-month follow-up (Spector et al. 1996).

A multipurpose, six-month exercise program combined submaximal quadriceps strengthening, bicycle aerobics, and a high-repetition routine for all the major muscle groups, including the quadriceps (Ernstoff et al. 1996). Quadriceps strength averaged 60 percent of the controls'. No fatigue monitoring was identified. The results identified no change in average quadriceps strength, though the weaker leg showed improved endurance.

Muscle biopsies showed mixed results. Among the six polio survivors in the intense program, two displayed only fibrosis (muscle loss?), two showed no change, and two exhibited further hypertrophy. In the multipurpose program, two individuals showed a loss of both strength and fiber area. None of the muscle fibers in the preexercise biopsies was described as atrophic. Biochemical study of the muscle biopsy samples displayed no short-term injury.

The outcomes of these studies indicate that polio survivors with adequate strength can engage in exercise if it is not overly vigorous, if the protocol is designed to avoid fatigue, and if the subject's lifestyle permits the added challenge. Certainly those who indulge in resistive exercise programs must carefully monitor the daily effects for signs of overuse injury. Countering the optimistic outcomes of these studies is Grimby's finding that the polio survivor with the greatest muscle fiber hypertrophy also had experienced the most strength loss over the preceding eight years (Grimby et al. 1998). All of the tissue studies focused on the muscle, yet the worrisome pathology is axon sprout destruction and secondary motor unit loss. There is no graded measure of this pathology other than muscle strength changes. MRI displays only the areas of gross loss. Macro EMG identifies motor unit size but not a muscle's total composition.

With the muscle biopsies consistently showing preexisting hypertrophy and little or no subsequent gain, why subject symptomatic polio survivors to the neuronal strain of intense exercise? The mechanics of living impose their own exercise demands. My rule is that a person can engage in any activity that does not cause pain and fatigue lasting more than ten minutes. For the nonsymptomatic polio survivor, judicious exercise would be appropriate.

Bicycle aerobic exercise to enhance cardiovascular function can improve cardiopulmonary endurance to a limited extent. A 15 percent improvement in Vo2 max followed a thrice weekly sixteen-week program once the protocol was modified to accommodate the polio survivor's limited endurance (Jones et al. 1991). Exercise bouts began with two-minute session instead of the usual five minutes. Also, the workload should be reduced to 60 percent of the heart rate reserve rather than the customary 70 percent. A second bicycle aerobics program realized only a 4 percent gain. For both groups the therapeutic gain was a reduction in perceived exertion. Aerobic exercise uses the limbs to challenge the heart. The same precaution about muscle overuse must be practiced.

Stretching also is classified as an exercise. Maintaining full hip and knee extension, an erect trunk, and good shoulder external rotation is a valuable adjunct to function. Stretching the heel cord should be done cautiously, however, since slight tightness (ten degrees) can compensate for calf muscle weakness.

Orthoses and Assistive Devices

Joint and muscle pain, muscle weakness, fatigue, and limited function are the indications for prescribing mechanical support in patients disabled by poliomyelitis. In a group of eighty-one polio survivors with the complaints described above, the 42 percent who had an orthosis or walking aid prescribed reported an improved ability to walk, less overall pain, reduction in knee pain, and a greater perception of walking safety (Waring et al. 1989). Daily rather than sporadic use of their orthoses also reduced fatigue and weakness. Modern orthoses are made from polypropylene instead of metal and leather, so they fit better, weigh less, and are more cosmetically acceptable.

Ankle-foot orthoses, once most frequently prescribed for a drop foot, now are primarily needed to avoid quadriceps overuse by supplementing a weak calf with a dorsiflexion stop and free plantar flexion range (Perry and Clark 1997). A simple leaf spring is adequate for the isolated drop foot.

Knee-ankle-foot orthoses are of two types. For people with excessive hyperextension, an offset knee joint that limits the deformity yet allows sufficient back-knee for stance stability also retains free flexion in swing. The few patients with a combination of a flexion deformity and severe quadriceps weakness must continue with a locked knee joint, but the ankle joint described above will enhance stability.

Crutches are the source of support for weak hip muscles. They also improve trunk stability. Reducing floor impact with crutches may relieve low back pain when a lumbar support is inadequate. Crutches let the arms share the task of weight bearing. This can place a strong burden on the shoulder muscles, however, since the shoulder joint is not designed for weight bearing. Rotator cuff tears are a not infrequent consequence of longtime use of crutches.

Scooters and wheelchairs are indicated when the arms, particularly the shoulders, cannot tolerate the strain of weight bearing. Manual wheelchairs also stress the shoulders. Consequently, powered chairs are indicated when neither the shoulders nor the legs can meet the demands of walking.

It is difficult for the polio survivor who escaped orthoses in the acute polio episode or who managed to discard them during convalescence to accept such a recommendation now. All such aids are visible signs of disability, and many of today's patients have managed to hide their impairment. Even a change in orthotic design can be disturbing. For both situations, a sympathetic and careful explanation of the postpolio pathology and the mechanics of the recommended device generally leads to acceptance, if not at first, by the next visit or so.

Pain Management

Postpolio pain is a sign of injury from overuse. The appropriate therapeutic answer is to reduce the strain by lifestyle modification, supplemented by mechanical aids as indicated. Since the first tissue reaction to overuse is inflammation, anti-inflammatory medication also is logical. But simple pain medicines merely mask the pain and allow polio survivors to continue their stressful activity.

When other measures have failed, a surgical procedure to correct a functionally obstructive or painful deformity can be very beneficial. Joint replacement for the painful hip or knee also is appropriate if the controlling muscles have at least grade 3+ strength.

Summary

After their acute polio episode, most polio survivors had some residual paresis, but with clever coping they successfully reentered society. Approximately thirty years later, a significant number of them are experiencing new muscle weakness, fatigue, muscle and joint pain, and loss of function. This was not originally anticipated, and the cause was not evident. New awareness of previous research on the pathology and healing course of acute polio and new research on the late effects of polio have identified a logical therapeutic course for the postpolio syndrome. The cause appears to be an overlooked neural mechanism of axon sprouting that restored significant muscle function as part of the acute healing process. Unfortunately, these sprouts now are failing from years of overuse. The muscle involved also has become less efficient. Function can be preserved by avoiding overuse, by lifestyle modification, and by selected mechanical aids. The indications for exercise are controversial.

REFERENCES

Agre, J. C., and Rodriguez, A. A. 1990. Neuromuscular function: Comparison of symptomatic and asymptomatic polio subjects to control subjects. *Archives of Physical Medicine and Rehabilitation* 71:545–51.

Bach, J. R., and Alba, A. S. 2001. Pulmonary dysfunction and sleep disordered breathing as post-polio sequelae: Evaluation and management. *Orthopedics* 14:1329–37.

Berlly, M. H., Strauser, W. W., and Hall, K. M. 1991. Fatigue in postpolio syndrome. *Archives of Physical Medicine and Rehabilitation* 72:115–18.

Bodian, D. 1949. Histopathologic basis of clinical findings in poliomyelitis. *American Journal of Medicine* 6:563–78.

Bodian, D. 1985. Motoneuron disease and recovery in experimental poliomyelitis. In *Late effects of poliomyelitis*, ed. L. S. Halstead and D. O. Weichers, 45–55. Miami: Symposia Foundation.

Bruno, R. L., Cohen, J. M., Galski, T., and Frick, N. M. 1994. The neuroanatomy of post-polio fatigue. *Archives of Physical Medicine and Rehabilitation* 75:498–504.

Edwards, G. B., Clark, W. H., and Drake, R. M., eds. 1958. *Poliomyelitis in California during the pre-vaccine period.* Berkeley: California State Department of Public Health.

Ernstoff, B., Wetterqvist, H., Kvist, H., and Grimby, G. 1996. Endurance training effect on individuals with postpoliomyelitis. *Archives of Physical Medicine and Rehabilitation* 77:843–48.

Feldman, R. M., and Soskolne, C. L. 1987. The use of nonfatiguing strengthening exercises in post-polio syndrome. In *Research and clinical aspects of the late effects of poliomyelitis*, ed. L. S. Halstead and D. O. Weichers, 335–41. White Plains, N.Y.: March of Dimes Birth Defects Foundation.

Grimby, G., Stalsberg, E., Sandberg, A., and Sunnerhagen, K. S. 1998. An 8-year longitudinal study of muscle strength, muscle fiber size and dynamic electromyogram in individuals with late polio. *Muscle and Nerve* 21:1428–37.

Guyton, A. C. 1971. The reticular activating system: Wakefulness, sleep, attention, brain waves and epilepsy. In *Textbook of medical physiology*, ed. A. C. Guyton, 705–15. Philadelphia: W. B. Saunders.

Halstead, L. S., and Rossi, C. D. 1985. New problems in old polio patients: Results of a survey of 539 polio survivors. *Orthopedics* 8:845–50.

Jones, D. R., Speier, J., Canine, K., Owen, R., and Stull, G. A. 1991. Cardiorespiratory responses to aerobic training by patients with postpoliomyelitis sequelae. *Journal of the American Medical Association* 261:3255–58.

Kemp, B. J., Adams, B. M., and Campbell, M. L. 1997. Depression and life satisfaction in aging polio survivors versus age-matched controls: Relation to postpolio syndrome, family functioning, and attitude toward disability. *Archives of Physical Medicine and Rehabilitation* 78:187–92.

Klein, M. G., Whyte, J., Keenan, M. A., and Esquenazi, A. 2000. Changes in strength over time among polio survivors. *Archives of Physical Medicine and Rehabilitation* 81:1059–64.

McNeal, D. R., Somerville, N. J., and Wilson, D. J. 1999. Work problems and accommodations reported by persons who are postpolio or have a spinal cord injury. *Assistive Technology* 11:137–57.

Mulroy, S. J., Lassen, K. D., Chambers, S. H., and Perry, J. 1997. The ability of male and female clinicians to effectively test knee extension strength using manual muscle testing. *Journal of Orthopedic Sports Physical Therapy* 26:192–99.

Patcher, B. R., and Eberstein, A. 1995. Rat model of the reinnervated motor unit: Relevance to the post-polio syndrome. *Annals of the New York Academy of Sciences* 753:158–66.

Peach, P. E., and Olejnik, S. 1991. Effect of treatment and noncompliance on post-polio sequelae. *Orthopedics* 14:1199–1203.

Perry, J., Barnes, G., and Gronley, J. K. 1988. The postpolio syndrome: An overuse phenomenon. *Clinical Orthopaedics and Related Research* 233:145–62.

Perry, J., and Clark, D. 1997. Biomechanical abnormalities of post-polio patients and the implications for orthotic management. *NeuroRehabilitation* 8:119–38.

Perry, J., and Fleming, C. 1985. Polio: Long-term problems. *Orthopedics* 8:877–81.

Ramlow, J., Alexander, M., LaPorte, R., and Kaufmann, C. 1992. Epidemiology of the post-polio syndrome. *American Journal of Epidemiology* 136:769–85.

Sharrard, W. J. 1955. Muscle recovery in poliomyelitis. *Journal of Bone and Joint Surgery* 37B:63–79.

Silbergleit, A. K., Waring, W. P., and Sullivan, M. J. 1991. Evaluation, treatment, and follow-up results of post polio patients with dysphagia. *Otolaryngology—Head and Neck Surgery* 104:333–38.

Sivakumar, K., Sinnwell, T., Yildiz, E., McLaughlin, A., and Dalakas, M. C. 1995. Study of fatigue in muscles of patients with post-polio syndrome by *in vivo* [^{31}P]magnetic resonance spectroscopy. *Annals of the New York Academy of Sciences* 753:397–401.

Spector, S. A., Gordon, P. L., Feuerstein, I. M., Sivakumar, K., Hurley, B. F., and Dalakas, M. C. 1996. Strength gains without muscle injury after strength training in patients with postpolio muscular atrophy. *Muscle and Nerve* 19:1282–90.

Spencer, W. A. 1954. *The treatment of acute poliomyelitis.* Springfield, Ill.: C. C. Thomas.

Sunnerhagen, K. S., Carlsson, U., Sandberg, A., Stalberg, E., Hedberg, M., and Grimby, G. 2000. Electrophysiologic evaluation of muscle fatigue development and recovery in late polio. *Archives of Physical Medicine and Rehabilitation* 81:770–76.

Tollback, A., Soderlund, V., Jakobsson, F., Fransson, A., Borg, K., and Borg, J. 1996. Magnetic resonance imaging of lower extremity muscles and isokinetic strength in foot dorsiflexors in patients with prior polio. *Scandinavian Journal of Rehabilitation Medicine* 28:115–23.

Waring, W. P., Maynard, F., Grady, W., Grady, R., and Boyles, C. 1989. Influence of appropriate lower extremity orthotic management on ambulation, pain, and fatigue in a postpolio population. *Archives of Physical Medicine and Rehabilitation* 70:371–75.

Weiss, P. and Edds, M. V. 1946. Spontaneous recovery of muscle following partial denervation. *American Journal of Physiology* 145:587–607.

Windebank, A. J., Litchy, W. J., and Daube, J. R. 1995. Prospective cohort study of polio survivors in Olmsted County, Minnesota. *Annals of the New York Academy of Sciences* 753:81–86.

Young, G. R. 1991. Energy conservation, occupational therapy, and the treatment of post-polio syndrome. *Orthopedics* 14:1233–39.

11

Aging with Cerebral Palsy

Kevin P. Murphy, M.D., and Patrick Michael Bliss, B.A., M.A.

The United Cerebral Palsy Association estimates that there are approximately 400,000 adults in the United States with cerebral palsy. This number is likely growing owing to advances in medical care, home support services, and the increased life expectancy of the general population. More than 90 percent of children with chronic illness or disability now survive into adulthood. Despite this, relatively little has been published regarding the general health and rehabilitation needs of adults with cerebral palsy. What has been published shows a wide disparity between medical and rehabilitation services for adults and those for children, with many more services available for children. This chapter will report on the current state of the field, including data on social and employment issues.

Cerebral palsy is a nonprogressive injury to the immature brain that occurs before age five. The condition is characterized by alterations in muscle tone, reflexes, and posture relating to the trunk and extremities. It can be associated with other conditions, such as seizure, learning disability, cognitive impairment, sensory deficiency, and growth problems. Causes of cerebral palsy may occur in prenatal, perinatal, or postnatal periods (Grether, Cummins, and Nelson 1993). Prenatal causes include intrauterine infections, toxic or teratogenic agents, and socioeconomic factors (trauma to the womb, lack of prenatal care, etc.). Neonatal causes include prematurity at less than thirty-two weeks gestation, low birthweight (less than 2,500 grams), a twin gestation (often one twin is affected and the other is not), and hypoxia (low oxygen to the brain). Postnatal causes include intracranial hemorrhage, infection, and coagulopathies (clotting disorders of the blood). Traumatic brain injury, even if it occurs before age five, does not cause cerebral palsy.

Spastic cerebral palsy is the most common form of the condition. Spasticity can be defined as an involuntary increase in muscle tone that is velocity dependent: the faster the limb is moved, the more tone and resistance are encountered; slower movements encounter less resistance. There are several types of spastic cerebral palsy: spastic quadriparesis (affecting all four limbs and the trunk), spastic diplegia (affecting the legs), and spastic hemiparesis (affecting one side, usually the right). Less common types of cerebral palsy produce hypotonia (low muscle tone), ataxia (poor balance and coordination), dyskinesia (movement disorder), and combinations of these impairments.

The overall incidence of cerebral palsy has not changed since the 1950s (Paneth and Kiely 1984). Marked improvements in perinatal care have likely prevented certain infants from developing cerebral palsy, while other infants have been saved from a likely death but develop cerebral palsy. This may explain why the incidence of the condition has been relatively unchanged over the past fifty years.

Management

Many recent advances have occurred in the treatment of cerebral palsy. These include marked advances in orthopedic surgery with computerized gait lab analysis, spasticity management with the use of botulinum toxin (Botox), and the intrathecal baclofen pump (ITB therapy). Computerized gait lab analysis is commonly used for children when decisions are being made about orthopedic surgery or equipment (Gage 1991). More adults with cerebral palsy are just beginning to use the gait lab, having gone without therapeutic orthopedic surgery in their childhood.

Physical therapists play a major role in collecting and analyzing the computerized data associated with functional and dysfunctional walking. The main problems that develop as people age into their thirties and forties are pain, excessive energy expenditure (fatigue), and falls. Excessive lumbosacral lordosis with crouch gait and anteverted hips (forward rotation of the femoral neck on the femoral shaft), creating toeing in, are common. Subsequent overuse syndromes with iliotibial band pain, patellofemoral dysfunction and malalignment (increased Q angles), and excessive external tibial torsion (rotation of the tibia outward) with painful midfoot breakage (severe pes valgus) are common impediments to long-term walking.

Adults with cerebral palsy are often fearful of major reconstructive surgery on their lower extremities, since it will temporarily take away their walking (approximately six to eight weeks of bony healing, with full recovery taking up to a year). They have struggled all their lives to maintain independence and functional walking, and the fear of losing that, even temporarily, may be overwhelming. Therapists play an important role during the preoperative period by providing strengthening exercises, patient education, and reassurance. The patient and the rehabilitation team members go through the surgery and year-long rehabilitation period together. Children typically make a full recovery from lower extremity reconstructive surgery in half the time it takes adults, usually about six months. Initial rehabilitation introduces weight bearing approximately two months after the operation, often in water. Dry-land therapy can begin within the first week after functional weight shifting and stepping have begun; adequate pain control is usually achieved with simple analgesics and modalities. The inpatient phase of rehabilitation usually takes four to six weeks, until the patient is able to return to an assisted home environment. Outpatient therapy typically continues for up to a year, with continued focus on strengthening and independent self-care skills.

Botox has been especially helpful in managing spasticity in specific muscle groups. The toxin blocks the release of acetylcholine at the neuromuscular junction, partially paralyzing the muscle for up to three months and thus allowing improved stretch and flexibility. For example, injecting Botox in an individual with toe walking or tight hamstrings relaxes the muscles to allow a more functional heel-toe gait pattern with improved step and stride length. Both occupational and physical therapists are required to stretch the soft tissues injected to promote muscle lengthening while also facilitating a functional home exercise program. Upper-extremity splinting is especially helpful in improving tissue length, particularly with the wrist, hand and digits, and across the elbow. Serial casting of the hands or feet may be very helpful following the Botox injection. Often the serial casts will be placed across the wrist and fingers, stretching them into comfortable extension, or across the ankle and foot, promoting the greatest tolerated dorsiflexion. Dynamic tone-reduction foot orthotics can be placed thereafter to encourage functional heel-toe walking and stability in gait, particularly over ground obstacles or on uneven surfaces. Botox injections do not have to be repeated every three months if the therapists and patient have succeeded in a good tissue lengthening program. Improved flexibility may be maintained long after the Botox neuroblockade has ceased.

When there is more diffuse muscle involvement, Botox injections may not be feasible. Instead, intrathecal baclofen is a better method to reduce spasticity. This involves inserting a catheter into the space around the spinal cord that contains the cerebral spinal fluid (CSF) and delivering the medication with a pump. If the baclofen allows muscle groups in the lower extremities to relax, functional movement improves and less caregiver assistance is needed. With less spasticity in the legs, it is much easier for a person with gross motor dependency to position, stand, step, and receive care.. It can also improve fluidity of gait in ambulatory adults, with decreased scissoring through the hips. Because the medication is delivered directly to the nerves, a much lower dose (by a factor of 1,000) is needed than with oral administration. Sedation and other serious systemic side effects are thus much reduced. Before the pump is implanted, a test dose is given by a single needle injection of between 50 and 100 mcg of baclofen into the spinal fluid. The therapy staff carefully measure spasticity reduction in both the upper and lower extremities. The peak reduction in spasticity is noted approximately four to six hours after the test dose is delivered. The Ashworth scale is frequently used to quantify spasticity (Penn et al. 1989). With this score, a measure of 1 is normal tone, 3 is marked increase in tone, and 5 is severe rigidity. Scores of 2 and 4 are shades in between. The spasticity must decrease at least one grade on the Ashworth scale after injection for a test dose to be considered positive. This indicates that the person is likely to benefit from the baclofen pump. Videotaping activities such as self-care, transfers, ambulation, and dressing is a helpful way to compare pre- and postoperative function, and it becomes an important part of the medical record.

Medical and Functional Issues

Primary, secondary, and associated conditions of cerebral palsy make up a large part of the medical needs for middle-aged and aging individuals. The primary condition of cerebral palsy has already been discussed. Secondary conditions are impairments, functional limitations, diseases, or injuries that occur as a result of or under the influence of the primary condition. Secondary conditions for adults with cerebral palsy often include pain, contractures, neurogenic bowel and bladder problems, gastroesophageal reflux (heartburn), poor dental hygiene, excessive joint wear and tear (possible early arthritis), and excessive menstrual cramping (Turk et al. 2001). Unlike secondary conditions, associated conditions are not a result of the cerebral palsy, yet they occur more often in people with cerebral palsy than in the general population. Associated conditions include seizures, learning disabilities, mental retardation, visual and hearing impairments, growth inequalities, and speech disorders, to name a few.

Secondary conditions also do not include comorbidities, which are other medical conditions unrelated to the primary physical condition. In other words, people with cerebral palsy can develop high blood pressure, diabetes mellitus, or cardiac disease (myocardial infarction) unrelated to their cerebral palsy at a frequency similar to that seen in the general population.

The lack of medical and rehabilitation services for adults with cerebral palsy has been well documented in the literature (Bax, Smyth, and Thomas 1988; Murphy, Molnar, and Lankasky 1995; Turk, Geremsky, and Rosenbaum 1997). General health care for adults with cerebral palsy seems to be adequate for acute illness but is woefully lacking for preventive medical care. Most adults go without routine primary care screening, including breast, pelvic, and prostate examinations, high blood pressure and cholesterol checks, and routine urine and bowel analyses.

We are just beginning to understand some of the difficulties in providing care for adults with cerebral palsy, including lack of space, staff, and equipment in the examination rooms, the need for increased time to communicate medical history and establish a physical diagnosis, and other socioeconomic factors. It can take an adult speaking with an augmentative communication device minutes or more just to answer a medical question in two or three simple sentences. Often adults with cerebral palsy are still treated as children by professional staff even though they may be their superiors in both intellect and maturity. The adult professional staff often resists seeing adults with cerebral palsy, since they consider the condition pediatric in nature and often lack appropriate training. Yet pediatric professionals are uncomfortable dealing with adult patients. Adults with cerebral palsy often fall into a gap of medical care where almost no medical professionals feel comfortable dealing with their conditions or comorbidities.

Figure 11.1 displays an example of arthritis in a forty-two-year-old man with

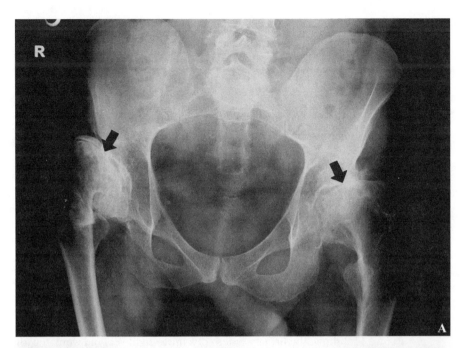

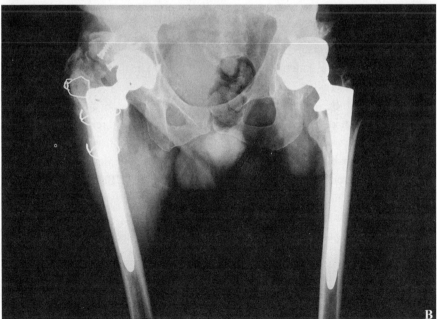

Figure 11.1. Arthritic formation in man with cerebal palsy before and after bilateral hip replacement.

cerebral palsy, spastic diplegic type. He had severe arthritis in both hips associated with chronic dislocations and pain. He could walk only a few feet before he had to stop because of pain. He was felt to be an excellent candidate for bilateral total hip arthroplasties. The adult orthopedic surgeon was uncomfortable operating on a person with cerebral palsy, a condition with which he had almost no experience. The pediatric orthopedist was uncomfortable operating on an adult needing artificial hips, a procedure with which he had limited experience. After some discussion, the two surgeons agreed to work together, and the surgery was successful. Postoperatively, the adult rehabilitation team members were concerned because they had not cared for many people with cerebral palsy. The interdisciplinary team meeting focused on the common principles of spasticity management, wound healing, and the postoperative total hip arthroplasty protocol of care. Emphasizing common rehabilitation principles well known to the staff made the cerebral palsy factor less of an issue. The subsequent rehabilitation outcome was beyond all expectations, and this adult is now walking more than a mile independently with his hips essentially pain-free.

Figure 11.2 shows the urinary system of a thirty-eight-year-old woman with cerebral palsy who has marked spastic quadriparesis. She was living in a group home, being treated by her family physician for kidney stones and hypertension. Her doctor believed that her urinary incontinence and difficulty voiding were simply consequences of the cerebral palsy. The therapy and nursing staff thought otherwise. The physical therapist was concerned about excessive spasticity in the trunk, lower extremities, and pelvic floor musculature. The nursing staff knew that the patient was quite capable and refused to accept incontinence as a way of life. This led to a group home team meeting and a subsequent rehabilitation consult. Computerized urodynamics revealed a spastic pelvic floor outlet obstruction (tight urinary sphincter). Because the sphincter was not opening well, the urine was refluxing into the kidneys, resulting in stone formation and bleeding. After placement of a suprapubic urinary catheter, providing adequate drainage of the bladder, the bleeding resolved, the kidney stones went away, and her blood pressure began to normalize. With this improvement in her health status the spasticity also decreased to very manageable levels. This case example underlines the importance of therapy and nursing advocacy for the patient while at the same time demonstrating how spasticity affects other body systems and vice versa. In this situation the pri-

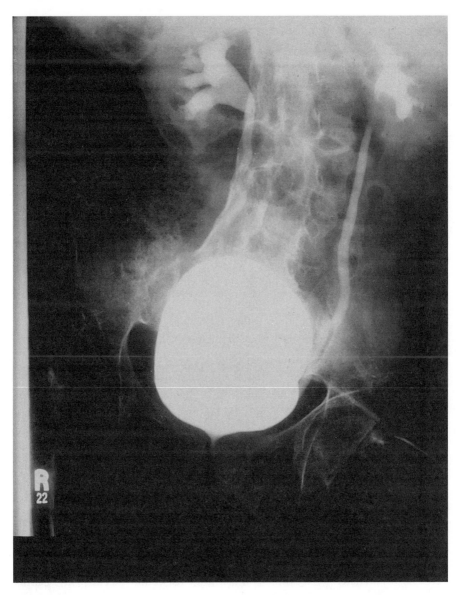

Figure 11.2. Urinary system of thirty-eight-year-old woman with cerebral palsy and incontinence.

mary condition of cerebral palsy with spasticity was causing secondary conditions of urinary obstruction and high blood pressure.

Data from the University of California at Riverside provide additional cause for concern (Singer, Strauss, and Shavelle 1998; Strauss and Shavelle 1998; Strauss, Cable, and Shavelle 1999). Excess standardized mortality ratios (SMR) were identified for adults with cerebral palsy. Specifically, mortality from breast cancer was three times that of the general population, suggesting poor detection or treatment or both. Dramatic SMR elevations were noted, with excessive deaths due to brain cancer, trauma, and diseases of the circulatory and digestive systems. Causes of trauma-related deaths included drowning and being hit by motor vehicles. This again raises concerns regarding the mobility of adults with cerebral palsy as they age. Physical therapists have a major role in helping them achieve safe and functional mobility, including transfers and walking, and manual and powered wheelchairs, and in preventing falls. Community access and efficient mobility in the workplace and other out-of-home environments are more than just a luxury. Lack of community access for adults with cerebral palsy can turn into a life-threatening situation. Further data from Strauss and Shavelle (1998) show that the lower the functional level, the higher the death rate. Survival of high-functioning adults was close to that of the general population. Excess mortality rates increase with age and show little difference between the sexes. It is encouraging that there are efforts by family practice physicians to organize around the care of adults with cerebral palsy. Rapp and Torres (2000) offered guidelines for general medical assessment and management. If implemented, these guidelines may result in decreased mortality ratios among this population with further understanding of secondary and associated conditions and comorbidities.

Rehabilitation needs require further study, because most adults report an almost total lack of professional service. For most people, durable medical equipment such as wheelchairs, braces, and gait aids is either lacking or seriously outdated. Excessive contractures, back and neck pain, spasms, scoliosis, shoulder dislocations and rotator cuff tears, internal derangement of knees (cartilage or ligament disruption), and carpal tunnel syndrome, to name a few, are frequent problems. Adult physical therapists may be uncomfortable seeing an adult patient with cerebral palsy and a yet-to-be-diagnosed rotator cuff tear. Often they see only the cerebral palsy, making diagnosis and treatment more difficult. Similarly, the pediatric therapist evaluating the same patient recognizes the condition of cerebral palsy well but knows little about the current diagnosis and treatment of shoulder pain in adults. A thirty-two-year-old woman with cerebral palsy having spasticity and dyskinesia came to our office practice. Her right knee was locking, with give-way weakness and deteriorating gait. She had seen numerous sports medicine doctors and an adult orthopedist, all of whom said that nothing further could be done and that gait deterioration was to be expected with cerebral palsy. An MRI scan showed a medial meniscus (posterior horn) with a partial tear. The adult orthopedist was encouraged toward arthroscopic surgical interventions to shave the meniscus and smooth out the joint surface. After the surgery, rehabilitation was rapid. Weight bearing occurred on the first postoperative day, with spasticity controlled by mild analgesics and low-dose diazepam. The principles of PRICE (protection, rest, ice, compression, elevation) were used with hydrotherapy the first couple of days. Once again, focusing on the common principles of care for patients following knee arthroscopy with minor adjustments for managing spasticity made the cerebral palsy factor less of an issue. This woman is now walking independently for long distances (more than a mile) with a stable knee and no pain. It is very easy for medical professionals (particularly physicians) to blame illness or the deterioration of function on the cerebral palsy without looking for other etiologies. We hope that with further collaboration, the gap in knowledge between adult and pediatric providers can be filled for the benefit of adults with cerebral palsy.

Employment Issues

With advances in technology, better home support services, legal mandates, and educational and environmental access, opportunities for adults with cerebral palsy seem to have improved. In the past, employment rates for people with mild to moderate disability were in the range of 10-15 percent. A recent study (Murphy, Molnar, and Lankasky 2000) of people in the community found that 53 percent of adults with cerebral palsy were competitively employed, including one-third of those with severe physical disability. More than 90 percent of the individuals with postsecondary education became competitively employed later in life. Sixty-five percent of them were self-supporting, and those who were not earned as much income as they could without losing disability benefits. Of the twenty-eight known nonambulatory people who

Table 11.1. Disability, employment, and annual rate of earnings: Individuals twenty-one to sixty-four years old

Disability	Total (thousands)	Employed (number/percentage)	Mean earnings ($) (value/standard error)
Mental retardation	746	220/29.5	7,545/1,292
Learning disability	605	166/27.5	10,450/2,305
Epilepsy	468	151/32.2	13,079/2,345
Head or spinal cord injury	699	289/41.3	17,212/2,165
Cerebral palsy	179	42/23.3	22,178/7,925
Visual impairment	1,280	627/49	23,844/2,397
Hearing impairment	1,873	1,409/75.2	31,650/3,176

Source: U.S. Census Bureau 1997, Survey of Income and Program Participation .

held competitive jobs, twenty-four used powered wheelchairs, and the other four had manual wheelchairs. It seemed quite clear to the authors that most nonambulatory adults needed powered wheelchairs to be competitive in employment.

Pel, Gillies, and Carss (1997) studied employment rates for people in Australia with physical disabilities. They found that 56 percent of those surveyed were employed either full time or part time. Computer skill level, training, and education were significant predictors of employment outcomes. The higher the level of computer skills and education, the higher the level of employment for adults with cerebral palsy and related conditions.

More representative results likely come from McNeil (1997), who examined data from the U.S. Census Bureau Survey of Income and Program Participation. Of the estimated 179,000 adults in the study with cerebral palsy, 23.3 percent were employed, with a median income of $17,623. Table 11.1 displays employment and average earnings across various disability groups. The United Cerebral Palsy Association, as of the year 2000, reported that the unemployment rate for all adults with cerebral palsy and related conditions was 75 percent versus 5 percent for able-bodied adults. According to the National Organization on Disability/Harris Survey of Americans with Disabilities (2000), people with disabilities are almost three times as likely as people without disabilities to live in poverty. Additional data from the Harris study indicate 22 percent of people with disabilities failed to complete high school compared with 9 percent of their able-bodied peers. However, improvements in employment, education, and related socioeconomic factors were noted over the past decade.

Social Issues

Issues of social concern were also reported in the California population according to Murphy, Molnar, and Lankasky (2000). In this study of community-dwelling adults with cerebral palsy, 84 percent felt that their parents overprotected them in childhood. They wished they had had more freedom for risk taking during their developmental years with respect to playground activities, peer interaction, and academic mainstreaming. Most felt that their mothers were the primary caregivers and wished their fathers had been more involved in their day-to-day routines. Sex education was virtually absent. Difficulty with meeting potential mates was a common frustration. Of the 6 percent of adults who were married, all but one were raising healthy, able-bodied children, and all had married someone who had cerebral palsy. Of those with severe speech deficits, over 90 percent had no functional augmentative communication device despite being judged capable of using one. More than 80 percent wished their physician knew more about cerebral palsy. They encouraged physicians to pay attention to their physical bodies but even more to the persons inside. Basic medical care was most frequently provided by chiropractors, followed by family practice physicians and other holistic paraprofessional medical staff.

Lifestyle studies on adults with cerebral palsy indicate clear differences from the able-bodied population. Steele et al. (2000) completed a health risk assessment on a large population of adults in Canada with cerebral palsy. They found that, compared with able-bodied peers, people with cerebral palsy made less use of tobacco, drugs, and alcohol. They also were less likely to exercise and more likely to watch television and eat junk food. The conclusions from the study were that health risk factors in adults with cerebral palsy may be markedly different from those of the general population. Heller, Factor, and Hahn (1999) examined the impact of moving adults with severe cerebral palsy out of nursing homes and into community-based settings. Assessments were made on movers and nonmovers, comparing variables concerning health and community functioning. Movers showed improved health status, mobility, and community functioning compared with nonmovers. Deinstitutionalizing had a positive effect on health status and socioeconomic variables.

Societal attitudes play a major role in the self-esteem and personhood of all people. In our society, individuals' worth is often judged by their ability to give back to the community economically, physically, socially, and intellectually. If people cannot "produce," then what is their use? Many people with cerebral palsy and related disabilities have had to face a society that tells them overtly or covertly, "You are not human enough." Over time, they may even start to believe some of these societal attitudes, thus taking on a much larger handicap than they might otherwise have. These false beliefs can follow the child into adulthood. Negative stereotypes of people with disabilities need to change toward a more positive and expansive definition of citizenship. This shift would include a focus on abilities more than disabilities and on alternative ways of giving back to the community. But in our opinion the primary impetus for change still resides in adults with cerebral palsy or related conditions, who need to choose positive and assertive ways of reacting to society and promoting healthy evolution in the surrounding community.

Transition Issues

The transition from childhood and adolescence into adulthood with a condition like cerebral palsy can be very difficult. Pediatric health care is basically child and family centered, with a focus on nurturing, growth, and development. Adult health care models are focused on patients who are often self-reliant, assertive, and well-informed decision makers, with family members assuming a more peripheral role. Multispecialty clinics are commonly available for children with cerebral palsy, spina bifida, or other developmental conditions. For the most part, similar multidisciplinary clinics are less available for adults. These differences make the transition to autonomy, independence, and community living more difficult. It is imperative that the child and adolescent with a disability learn healthy coping skills to be more capable in dealing with life as an adult. Perfectionism and control are two common coping mechanisms. Often adults with cerebral palsy will try to be exceptionally perfect in their dress, manner, and encounters in order to make up in some way for a negative perception of disability and handicap. Because they cannot always control their bodies with spasticity and movement disorders, they may attempt excessive control of their environments. It is important for health care providers to recognize and understand some of these coping mechanisms.

The Individuals with Disability Education Act requires that adolescent transition services be part of a teenager's individual education plan developed in the high schools before graduation (Spencer, Fife, and Ravinovich 1995). Input from academic therapy and nursing staff often proves critical, since educators have frequently received little if any training on the impairments or the medical conditions of their students. Such a transition plan is important for all teenagers although often lacking in a comprehensive way from institutions of secondary education. Spasticity management equipment, sports, and recreational medicine are life span issues along with other rehabilitation concerns requiring adult physiatric and therapy services. As the adult enters the workforce, carefully measured work stations need to be provided, along with appropriate job descriptions and performance expectations. This often involves physical and occupational therapy staff providing functional capacity assessments (FCAs), on-site ergonomic reviews, and work hardening programs. Mainstays of exercise in the adult with cerebral palsy include safe functional weight bearing with minimal pain, strengthening and flexibility routines, low-impact aerobics (often bicycle, tricycle, and swimming), and energy conservation principles. For people who are nonambulatory, standing tables with daily standing and lying prone can provide benefit. Often a nonambulatory adult with cerebral palsy can be standing or prone once or twice a day, thirty to sixty minutes at a time depending on tolerance and support staff. Customized prone lying wedges or contoured systems can make lying prone possible for almost any individual despite having scoliosis surgery with rods in place, severe hip flexion contractures, or tracheotomy and ventilation concerns. The therapy and nursing staff are integral in selecting equipment and helping with day-to-day exercise.

As parents age, they wonder who will care for their child with a disability when they no longer can. Lifelong planning is essential. Each plan must be individualized; there is no "one size fits all." Life span health care should also be the rule. By working with a fifty-year-old adult with cerebral palsy, we can often learn how best to care for the toddler, and vice versa. Insurance plans need to provide funding for services, equipment, and the basic dignities of life including communication, self-care, and mobility as aging continues. Life insurance can be difficult to find or afford for the adult with cerebral palsy, who may be married and raising a family. Estate planning can be complicated by false assumptions that physically impaired adults are not cognitively able to manage their own financial affairs.

Possibly the greatest transition that needs to occur is among our able-bodied selves. Expectations and attitudes toward children and adults with disabilities need to be elevated. For too long, barriers to successful transition for young people with disabilities have included low expectations by parents, teachers, health care providers, and other significant people in the community (O'Grady, Crain, and Kohn 1995; Blomquist et al. 1998). Positive change can be fueled by a new world of technology potentially available to all who can operate a switch. There seems no better time than now, the beginning of the third millennium, for such positive change to occur.

Summary

As the general population of the United States and other developed countries ages, so do people with cerebral palsy and related conditions. More than 90 percent of children with chronic illness or disability now survive into adulthood. The lack of specialty health care services and providers knowledgeable in the care of adults with childhood-onset conditions is a great concern. Pediatric providers are generally trained to treat patients through age eighteen and often know little about aging and acquired adult conditions. Adult health care providers are generally not trained in specialty conditions of childhood onset. For this reason, after age eighteen adults with cerebral palsy frequently find no health care professionals to provide service. Therapists, nursing staff, physicians, and related health care paraprofessionals can do much if given proper training in the health care of adults with cerebral palsy and their primary, secondary, and associated conditions. Secondary conditions seem most important, since they often can be prevented with appropriate intervention. Attitudes and expectations for adults with disabilities need to be elevated. Because of the advances in technology and computer service, state and federal legislation, academic mainstreaming, and community access, even those with the most severe physical disabilities can now be employed and living in an independent community home Despite these advances, much progress is still needed. It should be clear to all able-bodied people that we are simply one accident away from requiring the same services and equipment as those with cerebral palsy and related conditions. By our taking a personal interest in adults with cerebral palsy, maximal progress can be realized in the medical care and rehabilitation of this special population.

REFERENCES

Bax, M. C. O., Smyth, D. P. L., and Thomas, A. P. 1988. Health care of physically handicapped young adults. *British Medical Journal* 296:1153–55.

Blomquist, K. B., Brown, G., Peersen, A., and Presler, E. P. 1998. Transitioning to independence: Challenges for young people with disabilities and their caregivers. *Orthopedic Nursing* 17 (3): 27–35.

Gage, J. R. 1991. *Gait analysis in cerebral palsy.* Clinics in Developmental Medicine, no. 121. New York: Cambridge University Press.

Grether, J. K., Cummins, S. K., and Nelson, K. B. 1993. The California cerebral palsy project. *Pediatric Perinatal Epidemiology* 6:339.

Heller, T., Factor, A. R., and Hahn, J. E. 1999. Residential transitions from nursing homes for adults with cerebral palsy. *Disability and Rehabilitation* 21 (5–6): 277–83.

McNeil, J. M. 1997. *Population reports in survey of income and program participation.* Washington, D.C.: Economics and Statistics Administration, U.S. Bureau of Census.

Murphy, K. P., Molnar, G. E., and Lankasky, K. 1995. Medical and functional status of adults with cerebral palsy. *Developmental Medicine and Child Neurology* 37:1075–84.

Murphy, K. P., Molnar, G. E., and Lankasky, K. 2000. Employment and social issues in adults with cerebral palsy. *Archives of Physical Medicine and Rehabilitation* 81:807–11.

National Organization on Disability/Harris Survey of Americans with Disabilities. 2000. Study no. 12384. Sponsor AETNA Inc. and the JM Foundation. Harris Interactive, 111 Fifth Ave., New York, N.Y., 10003.

O'Grady, R. S., Crain, L. S., and Kohn, J. 1995. The prediction of long term functional outcomes of children with cerebral palsy. *Developmental Medicine and Child Neurology* 37:997–1005.

Paneth, N., and Kiely, J. 1984. The frequency of cerebral palsy. In *The epidemiology of cerebral palsies,* ed. F. Stanley and E. Alberman. Clinics in Developmental Medicine. Philadelphia: J. B. Lippincott.

Pel, S. D., Gillies, R. M., and Carss, M. 1997. Relationship between use of technology and employment rates of people with physical disabilities in Australia: Implications for education and training programmes. *Disability and Rehabilitation* 19 (8): 332–38.

Penn, R. D., Savoy S. M., Corcos, D., Latash, M., Gottlieb G., Parke B., and Kroin J. S. 1989. Intrathecal baclofen for severe spinal spasticity. *New England Journal of Medicine* 320:1517–21.

Rapp, C. E., and Torres, M. M. 2000. The adult with cerebral palsy. *Archives of Family Medicine* 9:466-72.

Singer, R. B., Strauss, D., and Shavelle, R. 1998. Comparative mortality in cerebral palsy patients in California, 1980-1996. *Journal of Insurance Medicine* 30:240–46.

Spencer, C. H., Fife, R. Z., and Ravinovich, C. E. 1995. The school experience of children with arthritis: Coping in the 1990's and transition into adulthood. *Pediatric Clinics of North America* 12:1285–98.

Steele, C., Kalnins, I., Bortolussi, J., Jutai, J., and Biggar, D. 2000. The American Academy for Cerebral Palsy and Developmental Medicine (AACPDM) 2000. Meeting abstracts.

Health risks of adolescents with physical disabilities. *Developmental Medicine and Child Neurology* 42 (Suppl. 83): 15–16.

Strauss, D., Cable, W., and Shavelle, R. 1999. Causes of excess mortality in cerebral palsy. *Developmental Medicine and Child Neurology* 41:580–85.

Strauss, D., and Shavelle, R. 1998. Life expectancy of adults with cerebral palsy. *Developmental Medicine and Child Neurology* 40:367–75.

Turk, M. A., Geremsky, C. A., and Rosenbaum, P. F. 1997. Secondary conditions of adults with cerebral palsy (final report). Health Science Center at Syracuse, New York, Centers for Disease Control and Prevention: R04/CCR 208516.

Turk, M. A., Scandale, J., Rosenbaum, P. F., and Weber, R. J. 2001. The health of women with cerebral palsy. *Physical Medicine and Rehabilitation Clinics of North America* 12 (1): 153–68.

12

Aging with Developmental Disabilities

Emerging Models for Promoting Health, Independence, and Quality of Life

Tamar Heller, Ph.D.

I just want what most people do: a living wage, a meaningful social life, a few good laughs, and the means to get around.
—Fifty-year-old man with cerebral palsy

In the past decade there have been major shifts in approaches to supporting adults with developmental disabilities and their families as they age. These shifts include greater inclusion in the community, more person-centered approaches that respect personal choices and address quality of life, and supports provided in the natural context in which people live, work, and play. This chapter addresses aging of people with developmental disabilities using a model of successful aging that emphasizes supports. Second, it presents innovative policies and programs that support health promotion, family caregiving and future planning, independence in work, home, and community settings, and greater self-determination.

Conceptual Model

The model of successful aging used is an adaptation of the supports-outcome model inherent in the latest definition of intellectual disabilities (American Association on Mental Retardation 1992) and an adaptation of the successful aging model popular in the gerontological literature. The supports-outcomes model of successful aging emphasizes the primacy of the environment and individualized supports in influencing outcomes for older adults. Outcomes of successful aging are independence, high quality of life, enhanced physical and emotional well-being, and full inclusion in the community. This definition includes the concepts of maintaining and enhancing independence, well-being, and perceived quality of life, including life satisfaction, goal attainment, and autonomy.

How successfully individuals age depends on the following things: capabilities, including intellectual level and adaptive behavior; environment, including home, work, and other community environments; physical and emotional health; physical functioning; and the amount and kind of support they receive. Overall functioning results from the interaction of people's capabilities, their environments, and the type and extent of support provided. Capabilities are general competence and attributes that enable individuals to function in society. Older adults with developmental disabilities experience differential rates of health and age-related changes in physical and mental health, most typically a decline. Since adults with some developmental disabilities (Down syndrome, cerebral palsy) undergo earlier age-related declines, much of the research includes people who are middle aged or older (at least thirty years old).

The environment comprises the demands and constraints of specific situations. Positive environments foster the individual's growth, development, and well-being in specific work, home, and community settings. For those with developmental disabilities, these positive environments constitute settings that are typical of their age peers and that are appropriate for their sociocultural background. Desirable environments have three major characteristics: they offer opportunities for fulfilling the person's needs; they foster well-being in physical, social, material and cognitive life areas; and they promote a sense of stability, predictability, and control. As a person ages these environments also undergo changes. For example, people with a developmental disability may move out of the family home when a parent dies or is too ill to provide care or retires from work because of age-related functional losses. People with developmental disabilities differ in the nature, extent, and severity of their functional limitations, often because of the demands and constraints of their environment and the presence or absence of supports.

This model emphasizes how support influence both functional and social outcomes of aging. Support can come from a number of resources, including other people, technology, and services. Supportive resources could be grouped

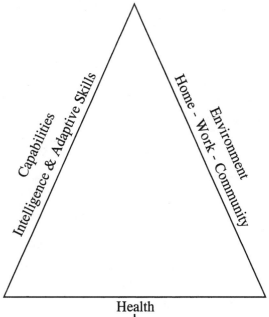

Health
↓
Functioning
↓ ↑
Supports

- friendships with family & friends
- financial planning
- behavioral & emotional support
- in-home living assistance
- community access & use
- health promotion & care

↓

Outcomes of Successful Aging

- independence & quality of life
- enhanced physical & emotional well-being
- full community inclusion

Figure 12.1. A model of successful aging.

around seven key areas: companionship from family and friends; financial planning; employee assistance; emotional and behavioral support; in-home living assistance; community access and use; and health promotion and care. These supports fluctuate throughout the life span. Often older adults receive fewer services than children and younger adults with developmental disabilities, since there are few mandates for adult services (see fig. 12.1).

To understand the types of supports needed to promote the successful aging of adults with developmental disabilities, this chapter will discuss demographic trends, age-related health changes, family context, and the nature of the service system in this population.

Demographics of Older People with Developmental Disabilities

The needs of older adults with developmental disabilities are gaining increased attention as that population continues to grow and its members become more visible in their communities. There are an estimated 526,000 adults sixty and older with intellectual disabilities and other developmental disabilities, and by 2030 that number will triple to more than 1.5 million. The life expectancy and age-related medical conditions of adults with developmental disabilities are similar to those of the general population unless they have severe levels of cognitive impairment, Down syndrome, cerebral palsy, or multiple disabilities. As with the general population, longevity among adults with developmental disabilities has increased considerably over the past fifty years. Reports show that the mean age at death now ranges from the late fifties for adults with Down syndrome to the middle sixties for adults with other intellectual disabilities (Janicki et al. 1999). The growing number of older adults with developmental disabilities will increase the need for services and supports that enable them to maintain functioning and continue to live as independently as possible, whether with family or in other residential settings.

Health Status and Health Promotion

Like the general population, adults with developmental disabilities are at risk for chronic medical conditions as they age, including cardiovascular disease, cancer, cerebrovascular disease, lung conditions, and diabetes. The prevalence of these diseases varies by the level of intellectual disability and the setting in which people live. For example, people with more severe intellectual disabilities who live in institutions are more likely to have respiratory conditions than those with less severe cognitive impairments (Horowitz et al. 2000). As they age, adults with developmental disabilities often develop secondary conditions caused by their disabilities. There is some evidence that people with a lifelong history of certain medications (e.g., psychotropics, antiseizure) have a higher risk of developing secondary health problems (e.g., osteoporosis, tardive dyskinesia; Adlin 1993). People with Down syndrome have a higher prevalence of Alzheimer disease at an earlier age than the general population (Janicki et al. 1996). Other health problems that adults with Down syndrome experience sooner than the general population include hypothyroidism, diabetes, cardiovascular disease, and sleep apnea (Chicoine, Rubin, and McGuire 1997; Horowitz et al. 2000). They also undergo other age-related declines earlier, such as sensory losses (Flax and Luchterhand 1996), adaptive behavior losses, and cognitive declines (Hawkins et al. 1997). There is some evidence that people with cerebral palsy also have earlier age-related difficulties with mobility (Mendelson and Heller 1997), incontinence, and swallowing (Arcand 1996).

Both environmental conditions and health habits affect health status. For example, when people with developmental disabilities were moved out of nursing homes into community residences, their health improved (Heller et al. 1998). Now the greater number of people aging in the community has raised concerns about defining models for dementia care, aiding "aging in place" for those with age-associated fragility and medical conditions, and providing specialized care related to terminal illnesses and age-associated conditions.

In addressing age-related changes among adults with developmental disabilities, clinicians and health care professionals need to be cognizant that their special health needs include the potential for earlier aging among some groups, the interaction of multiple drugs, and the impact of their long-term use. Because many people with developmental disabilities have long-term physical and cognitive impairments, age-related changes may be more difficult to detect. Also, communication difficulties make it harder to discover symptoms such as pain, fatigue, and discomfort. Hence it is important to conduct baseline assessments with ongoing follow-up. To improve communications, nonverbal modes such as pictures are often useful.

National health surveys reveal that the most common chronic health problems for adults with developmental disabilities are high blood pressure, osteoarthritis, and heart disease (Anderson 1997). For all these conditions, proper nutrition and exercise promote health and longevity. Among adults with intellectual disabilities, obesity and high cholesterol levels are more common than in the general population. This is particularly true for women and for adults living in independent settings (Rubin et al. 1998). Among adults with Down syndrome, Rubin et al. (1998) found that nearly half of the women and nearly one-third of the men were morbidly obese. The National Medical Expenditure Survey found that older adults with mental retardation living at home were less likely to quit smoking once they started and to exercise less frequently than other older adults (Anderson 1997). In addition to the negative effects on health, the high levels of obesity and the low levels of physical activity reported can create barriers to successful employment, participation in leisure activities, and activities of daily living.

Research studies of adults with Down syndrome (Heller, Hsieh, and Rimmer, in press) and adults with cerebral palsy (Heller et al., in press) have shown that the caregiver's attitude about exercising is a major determinant of how much people with developmental disabilities exercise. Interviews with adults with Down syndrome and their caregivers have shown that the major barriers to exercising are cost, transportation, and accessibility of fitness centers. In addition, there are psychosocial barriers, including perceived lack of time, energy, and health concerns (Heller et al., in press).

The University of Illinois at Chicago Center on Health Promotion Research for People with Disabilities and the Rehabilitation Research and Training Center (RRTC) on Aging with Developmental Disabilities have developed a health promotion program for middle-aged and older adults with developmental disabilities. It includes a twelve-week, three days per week center-based program of exercise, nutrition classes, and health behavior education. It also includes a caregiver education program. Its aims are to increase the physical functioning of these adults over the twelve weeks, increase their knowledge of healthy behaviors, and promote social and environmental supports for exercise adherence after the training ends. Its curriculum, *Exercise and Nutrition Health Education Curriculum for Adults with Developmental Disabilities* (Heller, Marks, and Ailey 2001), includes an instructor's guide and individualized student notebooks with their own pictures of themselves exercising. Pilot testing with the first twenty-nine participants indicated improvements in the participants' knowledge of the benefits of exercise, self-efficacy to perform exercises, greater life satisfaction, less loneliness, and fewer barriers to exercising. This research points to the importance of developing nutrition and fitness programs for adults with developmental disabilities and of improving accessibility of fitness centers in the community.

As people experience age-related declines in physical health, they are likely to require more health care. Major health gaps for adults with mental retardation living in the community include dental care (Jaskulski, Metzler, and Zierman 1990), home-based medical care, and gynecological care (Minihan and Dean 1990). Women with intellectual disabilities are less likely to receive Pap smears, breast exams, or mammography than the general population (Gill and Brown 2001). For older adults with developmental disabilities who are living in the community, inadequate health care is a major threat to their ability to stay independent. The key barriers to receiving adequate health care include uncoordinated systems of health care, health care providers' lack of training and knowledge, and poor ability of many adults with developmental disabilities to communicate their symptoms and to negotiate the health care system (Horowitz et al. 2000).

There is a need to educate not only health care professionals but also adults with developmental disabilities and their staff and family caregivers regarding age-related changes and ways to promote positive health behaviors. This can be done through specialized health education curricula, adapted fitness equipment, accessible fitness centers, and support staff involvement in adherence to health promotion programs and activities.

Family Caregiving and Future Planning

Families continue to be the primary providers of care. At least 60 percent of adults of all ages with intellectual disabilities live at home (Fujiura 1998), and many may not be known to the developmental disabilities service system. Among their family caregivers, more than 25 percent are themselves over age sixty (Braddock 1999). Because adults with developmental disabilities are living longer, families have a longer period of responsibility. Most parents providing care prefer having their son or daughter living with them after he or she reaches adulthood (Heller and Factor 1994). Families that want out-of-home placements often encounter long waiting lists or alternatives that are inadequate. Older families become less able to provide care as parents and siblings deal with their own aging, health problems, careers, and other caregiving responsibilities. Although families have strong preferences regarding the care of their relative when they can no longer provide it, fewer than half actually make a plan for the future (Heller and Factor 1991; Freedman, Krauss, and Seltzer 1997). How much families plan depends on socioeconomic resources, personal coping styles, and the options available in their communities (Heller and Factor 1991; Freedman, Krauss, and Seltzer 1997).

The increased longevity of adults with developmental disabilities has created a demand for services and special attention that most localities are ill prepared to address. Often there is conflict over which is the responsible service system—aging or developmental disabilities; who the primary client should be—the aging caregiver, the person with a developmental disability or the family; and what are appropriate service models—maintaining the family living situation, planning for transitions to out-of-home living, or promoting the independence of the person with a developmental disability. In addition, many older carergivers may avoid contact with formal service providers. The lack of attention by the formal service system and the reluctance of families to seek out assistance conspire to create crises for these families. When a caregiving parent dies or becomes too ill to continue care, formal agencies are likely to be approached to provide out-of-home care on an emergency basis. Prior engagement with families, planning for their needs, and cooperation among service agencies are more likely to yield less costly and less disruptive service options. The challenge is to determine how agencies mobilize to address the needs of such families. There are still many older parents who have had no contact with formal organizations and who are at risk owing to their own aging and the aging of their son or daughter with a developmental disability (McCallion and Tobin 1995). Also, families from cultural minorities who have a member with a lifelong disability frequently are underreported among formal service recipients and often not included in aging network services.

Parents have been an undeniable resource for the service systems, and parents who provide lifelong homes for their sons or daughters make a major contribution not only to their families but also to society. Families have considerable out-of-pocket expenses when an adult relative with developmental disabilities lives at home.

In one of the only studies that detailed families' cash expenditures (Fujiura, Roccoforte, and Braddock 1994), families spent an average of 20 percent of their pretax annual income on unreimbursed expenses for their adult relative. To maintain this living arrangement, parents report needs for respite services, case coordination, and transportation. Other unmet needs are for information regarding residential programs, financial plans, and guardianship and respite services (Heller and Factor 1993; Heller, Miller, and Hsieh 1999). While there has been an increase in funding for family support programs in the past ten years, these programs represent a small portion of spending for developmental disabilities services, accounting for only 2 percent of expenditures (Braddock et al. 1998), and many of these programs target only children. Most of the innovative family support programs include models of consumer control in which families determine how resources are spent. These are based on the premise that families usually know best what it takes to maintain their relative with a disability in the family home. They also acknowledge the importance of using the informal network, including relatives, neighbors, and friends, by allowing families to pay them for support services. To promote such flexibility, families receive cash subsidies to spend as they choose or within certain parameters or are given vouchers to acquire various supports. Most of the studies evaluating the impact of cash subsidies or vouchers for families have focused on families of children. Heller et al. (1999) conducted one of the few studies of a statewide family support program for adults with developmental disabilities. Compared with families who did not receive these services, participating families reported greater caregiving satisfaction and greater feelings of competence and efficacy in helping their relatives. Additional benefits included more community integration and improved interpersonal relations of adults with developmental disabilities, fewer unmet service needs, more satisfaction with services received, less need for out-of-home placement, and more legal and financial planning.

Several statewide and federal projects have sought to provide information and encouragement to families in making long-term plans. Examples include the Family Futures Planning Project in Rhode Island (Susa and Clark 1996), Planned Lifetime Advocacy Network in British Columbia (Etmanski 1997), Family-to-Family Project in Massachusetts (Community Service Reporter 1999), and the RRTC on Aging with Mental Retardation Multicultural Family Future Planning Project (Preston and Heller 1996). Each project differed in the families targeted, the curriculum and information provided, and the way that support was provided.

The Family Futures Planning Project in Rhode Island specifically targeted older family caregivers (Susa and Clark 1996). The ten-session curriculum included information on such topics as housing options, estate planning, and home- and community-based services. Other issues include caregivers' emotional and physical health and leisure activities. A paid facilitator helped families develop a plan and build a support network. The focus was on the family's needs rather than on the needs of the individual with an intellectual disability. The aging and developmental disabilities systems successfully collaborated in supporting families through the project. Only eighteen families participated, but because of the intimacy of the small groups, they were able to share experiences and provide support to one another. As part of this project families identified barriers to future planning and began to move ahead with making changes.

The Planned Lifetime Advocacy Network (PLAN), in British Columbia, is a family-operated nonprofit organization (Etmanski 1997). PLAN receives no government funding, but half of the funding comes directly from families. Hence it reaches only families who can afford membership. PLAN has developed a six-step guide to developing a personal future plan: clarifying your vision, building relationships, controlling the home environment, preparing for decision making, developing your will and estate plan, and securing your plan. PLAN provides many levels of support and services and uses mentor families, who attend meetings and visit other families, in addition to paid facilitators who help to develop a support network. Workshops and technical assistance are provided to families. Also, PLAN conducts systems advocacy through lobbying at the government level. The mission of PLAN is to provide a "lifetime commitment" to families and to help them create a secure future for their family member with a disability.

The Family-to-Family Project in Massachusetts targeted all families having a family member on the waiting list for residential services. The project developed eight Family-to-Family Support Centers across the state. The centers' activities varied. They included presentations on special needs trusts and wills, homeownership and consumer-controlled housing, circles of support, and presentations by self-advocates. A resource manual with information concerning funding sources, housing options, and legal issues was compiled and translated into several languages. Most of the sites conducted outreach to unserved families. Monthly parent groups were formed where participants shared support and exchanged information. Letters written by families and a state survey conducted by the project were sent to legislators in order to achieve systems advocacy.

The RRTC Multicultural Family Future Planning project conducted legal and financial training with 220 families at seventeen sites. One site included primarily African American families, and another site targeted Hispanic families. The training of family and staff members consisted of two-day training workshops conducted by a lawyer and a parent of an adult with an intellectual disability. In addition, case coordinators received training on ways to provide support and follow-up to families. Case coordinators conducted six months of follow-up.

Although most of these interventions did not report empirical results, anecdotal information suggests they had limited success in stimulating planning. The key initiatives have generally included a training component, but they vary in how much they use paid facilitators and other parents as mentors. None of the key projects included peer mentors or training for the person with an intellectual disability. While families generally note a high need for training about planning and rate such training very positively, they often do not follow up the training with concrete actions or plans. The Planned Advocacy and Network Project noted that only 5 percent of families who attended its training workshops actually made plans (Etmanski 1997). Similarly, six months after the RRTC legal and financial training, most families still had not made much progress in developing plans (Preston and Heller 1996). In our preliminary survey, most families said they intended to plan but felt they needed more support in dealing with the psychological issues and in negotiating the service system. Yet they rated these workshops very positively. The Family Futures Project in Rhode Island (Susa and Clark 1996), which included training and a paid service facilitator, reported that very few families made plans during the project's eighteen-month period, but that the project was successful in getting them to progress in the planning process. The PLAN project, which included training with family mentoring and ongoing support, reported more success in helping families plan when they sought the ongoing support from other families. The Massachusetts Family-to-Family Project was successful in setting up networks of families, with eight networking center around the state. Its major success was helping families on the waiting list for residential services learn from other families about ways to develop family-financed housing approaches and about ways to advocate for system change.

To better help families through the planning process, it is important to attend to the psychosocial issues that prevent them from making plans, to provide information on available supports to both the family caregivers and the person with a disability so that they can make informed choices, and to provide ongoing support. This support can include paid facilitators or mentoring by other families and people with disabilities who have gone through the process. In addition, families can be encouraged to think about their hopes for the future of their relative with a disability and to get involved in advocacy that can lead to systems change.

Maintaining Independence in Residential, Employment, and Community Settings

The nature and character of residential services for people with developmental disabilities have changed markedly over the past two decades. There has been a pronounced shift from large congregate settings to community living arrangements. Between 1977 and 1996, total public spending for community residential settings for fifteen or fewer people and nonresidential services increased sevenfold, from $2 billion to $14 billion in 1996 dollars. In contrast, public expenditures for congregate facilities for sixteen people or more have remained relatively stable, increasing slightly from $6.5 billion to just over $7 billion (Braddock et al. 1998). There also has been a trend toward small-scale settings. Fiscal year 1995 marked the first time individuals in settings of six people or fewer constituted the majority (51.8 percent) of individuals in mental retardation/developmental disability residential settings.

Despite these progressive changes, there is still a widespread shortage of housing. Over 80,000 adults with intellectual disabilities and other developmental disabilities are on waiting lists for residential services (Prouty and Lakin 1996). Several states have specific waiting list initiatives that are seeking to provide family-based supports, and more support housing to meet these demands. Major initiatives are under way in Massachusetts, Maryland, Pennsylvania, and New Jersey. For example, in Massachusetts, in addition to increasing expenditures for these services, the state has helped to foster family-to-family networks that offer peer support and information to families on the waiting list.

Several federal programs offer housing options for adults with intellectual disabilities, including the Housing and Community Development Act of 1987 (PL 100-142); the Stewart McKinney Homeless Assistance Act of 1987 (PL 100-77); the National Affordable Housing Act of 1990 (PL 101-402); the Farmers' Home Administration's Guaranteed Loan Program; and the Federal National Mortgage Association (Fannie Mae) (Stone 1994). However, owing to budget constraints, all federally subsidized housing serves fewer than one-third of all eligible applicants with and without disabilities (National Council on Disability 1996).

At present, more than 60 percent of people with intellectual disabilities live with their families (Fujiura 1998). The sizable projected increase in the number of older individuals over the next thirty years will fuel the demand for supports across residential settings. Adults with disabilities who live in out-of-home residences will need supports to "age in place," and those living at home with parents will need new options as they outlive their parents. The magnitude of the aging population suggests that supports in the natural home and family-financed housing will increase in importance in light of the dramatic shortage of publicly funded community living arrangements.

Most adults with developmental disabilities are not employed. Recent analyses of the Survey of Income and Program Participation indicated that fewer than 25 percent of adults with intellectual disabilities have jobs, and those who do earn half what the general population makes ($1,000 versus $2,000 per month) (Yamaki and Fujiura 1999). Older people with developmental disabilities are as diverse as the general population in their attitudes about retirement (Factor 1989). Many older adults prefer to continue working as long as possible, and many people in workshops would like to move to better paying jobs in the community (Factor 1989; Heller et al. 1996).

Supported employment provides an opportunity for people with developmental disabilities to earn significantly higher wages and to experience positive social interaction in the workplace. A consumer satisfaction study of 110 employees with developmental disabilities and other disabilities in Virginia revealed that participants were relatively young, with an average age of thirty-two (Kregel and Wehman 1996). Although little is known about access to supported employment initiatives for older people, studies of vocational opportunities for older workers with disabilities often show that they are the victims of age discrimination and institutional neglect. State vocational rehabilitation agencies often provide myriad resources for those workers with long-term work life potential but neglect older applicants. Thus, being an older adult with developmental disabilities can pose a considerable barrier to getting and keeping a job.

One major barrier to "aging in place" for people with developmental disabilities is a lack of access to personal assistance services, which are publicly funded in only fourteen states, with 12,220 people served (Braddock et al. 1998). Such services include personal care and homemaker or chore services provided in a variety of locations such as the home and work or recreational settings. The independent living model maintains that consumers should direct their own personal care when possible. This could include hiring, training, firing, supervising, and paying personal care assistants. This approach could result in more flexible, individualized services, cost savings, and better relations between providers and consumers. However, its success depends in part on consumers' capacity to direct the services, their training in managing services, and adequate monitoring of services. People with cognitive impairment may need more support and training in directing their services than people with other disabilities. For those with cognitive impairments, families often play a greater role in directing personal assistance services. Adults with developmental disabilities are seldom consulted about the type of services they want. Most of the decisions are made by parents (Heller, Miller, and Hsieh 1999). As more adults with developmental disabilities serve in leadership positions and provide greater input into the services they use, there will be a growing need for them to learn choice-making and leadership skills. We also need to develop ways to deliver support to older adults with cognitive disabilities and their families that better maintain their sense of autonomy and personal control.

Accommodating to Changing Needs through Assistive Technology

For older adults with developmental disabilities, age-related changes in health, social relationships, and cognitive functioning necessitate additional supports that help them maintain functioning and continue living as independently as possible, whether with family or in other residential settings. As functional limitations increase, so does the need for assistance with daily living skills. The need for ongoing personal care can preclude independent living, in some cases resulting in nursing home placement when neither family members nor community supports are available. Lack of independence can also prevent community integration by hindering an individual's ability to fully participate in vocational, social, and recreational activities. A synopsis of a series of White House Conference on Aging miniconferences for consumers with developmental disabilities reported that their major fear was being institutionalized and that their major unmet need was for in-home family supports that would enable them to live at home (Factor 1995). With advances in assistive technology and with supported living models that provide personal assistance or respite, in-home health, and homemaker services, it is possible to help people age in place, that is, continue living in their homes. However, we are only beginning to learn about approaches that are effective for this population.

There have been major technological advances in the field of rehabilitation that enable individuals to maintain or improve functional independence. In many cases appropriate assistive devices and strategies can overcome limitations in activities of daily living, communication, and mobility. The National Council on Disability (1993) found that for working-age people, assistive devices allowed 62 percent to depend less on family members and 58 percent to depend less on paid assistants. A demonstration project at the University of Illinois at Chicago's Assistive Technology Unit showed that providing assistive devices reduced public expenditures on homemaker services and Meals-on-Wheels in Chicago (Hedman 1996).

There are myriad examples of assistive technology that can aid in maintaining adaptive functioning in the face of age-related increases in impairment. For vision loss, examples include magnifiers, larger text screens, lights, and tactile cues. For hearing loss, in addition to hearing aids, tools include amplifiers, vibrating devices, microphones, devices to reduce background noise, visual cues, and signage. Mobility aids include canes, walkers, wheelchairs, and individualized seating and mobility adaptations. Examples of environmental accommodations include ramps, grab bars, and accessible toilets and showers.

Despite its value, many individuals with developmental disabilities who might benefit from assistive technology do not have all the equipment they need. A national survey conducted by Wehmeyer (1995) found that assistive technology was underused by people with intellectual disabilities, partly because fewer devices have been developed for cognitive impairments than for physical impairments. Second, even when devices are available, people with cognitive impairments have greater difficulty using them and understanding instructions regarding their use. Also, staff and families often are unaware of assistive technology, and funding for assessment and procurement of devices is insufficient. Several studies have begun to document the specific needs for and benefits of assistive technology for older adults with developmental disabilities.

Mendelson, Heller, and Factor (1995) found that among nursing home residents fewer then 15 percent with mobility impairments, 4 percent of those with communication limitation, and 6 percent of those with limitations in daily activities were using assistive devices. The types of equipment most needed by the residents were wheelchairs and seating systems. In a study focusing on older adults with cerebral palsy living in community settings, Mendelson and Heller (1997) found that residents of group homes used nearly twice as many assistive devices as residents of family homes, despite having similar needs for equipment. Lack of access to assistive devices among adults with cerebral palsy living at home placed them at a significant disadvantage in performing independent self-care and in community participation. The equipment used by group home residents was more often meant to increase individuals' functional abilities, while the equipment used by family home residents tended to reduce the burden on caregivers. These studies demonstrate the need to inform family members about assistive devices that could benefit their kin and to inform service providers and policymakers about the need for funding mechanisms that can provide assistive technology to individuals. Furthermore, in a follow-up study of this sample Hammel, Heller, and Ying (1998) found that the use of assistive technology increased adaptive functioning for the participants.

The challenge for the field is to continue developing assistive technology for people with developmental disabilities that will let them participate fully in the life of their community. This entails not only adequate assessment of functional impairments, but also assessments of the environmental context and ways to support the use of assistive technology where people live, work, and play. Therapists and other assistive technology specialists need first to be cognizant of patterns of age-related changes in various subgroups of this population and to understand the implications of these changes for daily roles and activities. They need to determine the type of intervention that is most likely to reduce stress and yet provide sufficient challenge to maintain optimal functioning. Involving both people with disabilities and their support givers (family and staff) in joint problem-solving strategies increases the likelihood of long-term and effective use of assistive technology and its fit with people's daily life patterns.

Self-Determination and Leadership

Over the past decade the self-advocacy movement for people with developmental disabilities has increased substantially; there are now more than one thousand chapters nationwide (Hayden and Senese 1996). Coupled with this movement there is a growing recognition that consumers need to have a part in developing, controlling, and monitoring the services they use. Throughout the United States, self-advocacy groups are instituting programs that give families and people with disabilities more choice and control over the services received. For example, the Robert Wood Johnson Foundation has funded self-determination initiatives for adults with developmental disabilities and their families in more than thirty states. However, older adults with developmental disabilities typically have had few opportunities for making choices and for self-determination in their lives. They also have little understanding of the concept of choice making (Heller, Pederson, and Miller 1996). An example of a curriculum that teaches aging concepts and choice-making skills is *Person-Centered Planning for Later Life: A Curriculum for Adults with Mental Retardation* (Sutton et al. 1993). Through this intervention we have been successful in teaching older adults with less severe developmental disabilities to understand the concept of choice making, to articulate their preferences, and to increase their daily choice making (Heller et al. 2000). One innovative approach has been the use of peer trainers. Adults with developmental disabilities can learn to be effective co-trainers and have helped increase the choice-making skills of other adults with developmental disabilities. In addition to serving as trainers, such adults are increasingly being called on to serve on boards and in other leadership positions. Pederson and Nelis (1997) noted that true partnership between people with developmental disabilities and members of decision-making groups involves three essential elements: sufficient training of people with developmental disabilities in assuming leadership roles, sufficient training of professionals and other committee members to share leadership, and sufficient ongoing support for people with developmental disabilities in leadership roles. In a study examining participation of adults with developmental disabilities in training, research, and leadership positions, Heller et al. (1996) found that major barriers to greater participation were difficulty in understanding the content of activities; socioemotional and self-respect issues, such as feeling that one's opinion was ignored; logistical difficulties, such as lack of transportation to meetings; and personal support difficulties, such as support workers who do not adequately help consumers.

Summary

This chapter has described some of the emerging models and programs to address the age-related changes of adults with developmental disabilities. We need to further develop public policies and interventions that increase health, promote work and home accommodations, help older adults age in place, and support family caregivers. To increase our understanding of the most effective interventions, we need more research that examines the processes and outcomes of various approaches and examines the impact of rapidly changing policies in health and long-term care.

REFERENCES

Adlin, M. 1993. Health care issues. In *Older adults with developmental disabilities: Optimizing choice and change*, ed. E. Sutton, A. Factor, B. Hawkins, T. Heller, and G. Seltzer, 49–60. Baltimore: Paul H. Brookes.

American Association on Mental Retardation. 1992. *Mental retardation: Definition, classification, and systems of supports*, 9th ed. Washington, D.C.: American Association on Mental Retardation.

Anderson, D. 1997. Health status and conditions of older adults with intellectual disabilities. Paper presented at the Eighth International Roundtable on Aging and Intellectual Disability, Chicago.

Arcand, M. 1996. Cerebral palsy and aging: A report to adults with cerebral palsy and their family. Madison: Wisconsin Council on Developmental Disabilities.

Braddock, D. 1999. Aging and developmental disabilities: Demographic and policy issues affecting American families. *Mental Retardation* 37:155–61.

Braddock, D., Hemp, R., Parish, S., and Westridge, J. 1998. *The state of the states in developmental disabilities*. 5th ed. Washington, D.C.: American Association on Mental Retardation.

Chicoine, B., Rubin, S., and McGuire, D. 1997. Health and psychosocial findings of the Adult Down Syndrome Center. Presentation at the International Roundtable on Aging and Intellectual Disability, Chicago.

Community Service Reporter. 1999. Family-to-Family project helps to reduce Massachusetts' waiting list. *Community Services Reporter*, May 1999, 4–5.

Etmanski, A., with Cammack V. and Collins J. 1997. *Safe and secure: Six steps to creating a personal future plan for people with disabilities*. Vancouver, B.C.: Planned Lifetime Advocacy Network.

Factor, A. 1989. *A statewide needs assessment of older persons with developmental disabilities in Illinois*. Chicago: University of Illinois at Chicago, Institute for the Study of Developmental Disabilities.

Factor, A. 1995. Reviewing the White House Conference on Aging and looking ahead. In *ADDvantage newsletter*. Chicago: Rehabilitation Research and Training Center on Aging with Mental Retardation, Institute on Disability and Human Development, University of Illinois at Chicago.

Flax, M. E., and Luchterhand, C. 1996. *Aging with developmental disabilities: Changes in vision*. Chicago: Arc and Rehabilitation Research and Training Center on Aging with Mental Retardation, Institute on Disability and Human Development, University of Illinois at Chicago.

Freedman, R. I., Krauss, M. W., and Seltzer, M. M. 1997. Aging parents' residential plans for adults children with mental retardation. *Mental Retardation* 35:114–23.

Fujiura, G. 1998. Demography of family households. *American Journal on Mental Retardation* 103:225–35.

Fujiura, G., Roccoforte, J., and Braddock, D. 1994. Cost of family care for adults with mental retardation and related developmental disabilities. *American Journal on Mental Retardation* 99:250–61.

Gill, C., and Brown, A. 2001. Overview of health issues of older women with intellectual disabilities. *Physical and Occupational Therapy in Geriatrics* 18:23–36.

Hammel, J., Heller, T., and Ying, G. 1998. Outcomes of assistive technology services and use by adults with developmental disabilities. *Proceedings of the Rehabilitation Engineering and Assistive Technology Society of North America Conference* (Minneapolis).

Hanson, D. 1992. The National Affordable Housing Act of 1990: Housing opportunities for people with disabilities. *Directions: Newsletter of the Illinois Planning Council on Developmental Disabilities.*

Hawkins, B. A., Eklund, S. J., Hsieh, C., and Ohlsen, C. T. 1997. Aging-related changes in persons with Down syndrome: Longitudinal findings. Paper presented at the Eighth International Roundtable on Aging and Intellectual Disability, Chicago.

Hayden, M. F., and Senese, D. 1996. *Self-advocacy groups: 1996 directory for North America.* Minneapolis: University of Minnesota, Research and Training Center in Community Living, Institute on Community Integration.

Hedman, G. 1996. The Assistive Technology Chicago Project. In *Proceedings of the RESNA Annual Conference*, 35–37. Arlington, Va.: RESNA Press.

Heller, T., and Factor, A. 1991. Permanency planning for adults with mental retardation living with family caregivers. *American Journal of Mental Retardation* 96:163–76.

Heller, T., and Factor, A. 1993. Aging family caregivers: Changes in burden and placement desire. *American Journal on Mental Retardation* 98:417–26.

Heller, T., and Factor, A. 1994. Facilitating future planning and transitions out of the home. In *Life-course perspectives on adulthood and old age*, ed. M. M. Seltzer, M. W., Krauss, and J. Janicki, 39–50. Monograph Series. Washington, D.C.: American Association on Mental Retardation.

Heller, T., Factor, A., Hsieh, K., and Hahn, J. 1998. The impact of transitions out of nursing homes and aging for adults with developmental disabilities. *American Journal on Mental Retardation* 103:236–48.

Heller, T., Hsieh, K., and Rimmer, J. In press. Barriers and supports for exercise among adults with Down syndrome. *Journal of Gerontological Social Work.*

Heller, T., Marks, B., and Ailey, S. 2001. *Exercise and nutrition health education curriculum for adults with developmental disabilities.* Chicago: Rehabilitation Research and Training Center on Aging with Developmental Disabilities, Department of Disability and Human Development, University of Illinois at Chicago.

Heller, T., Miller, A., and Hsieh, K. 1999. Impact of a consumer-directed family support program on adults with developmental disabilities and their family caregivers. *Family Relations* 48:419–27.

Heller, T., Miller, A., Sterns, H., and Hsieh, K. 2000. Later life planning: Promoting knowledge of options and choice-making. *Mental Retardation* 38:395–406.

Heller, T., Pederson, E. L., and Miller, A. B. 1996. Guidelines from the consumer: Improving consumer involvement in research and training for persons with mental retardation. *Mental Retardation* 34:141–48.

Heller, T., Sterns, H., Sutton, E., and Factor, A. 1996. Impact of person-centered later life planning training program for older adults with mental retardation. *Journal of Rehabilitation* 62:77–83.

Heller, T., Ying, G., Marks, B. A., and Rimmer, J. H. In press. Determinants of exercise participation in adults with cerebral palsy. *Journal of Public Health Nursing*.

Hodas, B. S. 1998. *The Housing and Community Development Act: A housing resource guide*. Glenside: Pennsylvania Self-Determination Housing Project.

Horowitz, S., Kerker, B., Owens, P., and Zigler, E. 2000. *The health status and needs of individuals with mental retardation*. New Haven: Yale University School of Medicine.

Janicki, M. P., Dalton, A. J., Henderson, C. M., and Davidson, P. W. 1999. Mortality and morbidity among older adults with intellectual disability: Health services considerations. *Disability and Rehabilitation* 21:284–94.

Janicki, M., Heller, T., Seltzer, G., and Hogg, J. 1996. Practice guidelines for the clinical assessment and care management of Alzheimer's disease and other dementias among adults with intellectual disability. *Journal of Intellectual Disability Research* 40:374–82.

Jaskulski, T., Metzler, C., and Zierman, S. A. 1990. *Forging a new era: The 1990 reports on people with developmental disabilities*. Washington, D.C.: National Association of Developmental Disabilities Councils.

Kregel, J., and Wehman, P. 1996. Supported employment research: Impacting the work outcomes of individuals with disabilities. In *Improving supported employment outcomes for individuals with the most severe disabilities newsletter*, ed. K. J. Inge. Richmond, Va.: Rehabilitation Research and Training Center at Virginia Commonwealth University.

Martinson, M. C., and Stone, J. A. 1992. *The Stewart B. McKinney Homeless Assistance Act: Models for interagency planning for long-term funding of small-scale community living options for older persons with developmental disabilities*. Lexington: Interdisciplinary Human Development Institute, University of Kentucky.

McCallion, P., and Tobin, S. S. 1995. Social worker orientations to permanency planning by older parents caring at home for sons and daughters with developmental disabilities. *Mental Retardation* 33:153–62.

Mendelson, L., and Heller, T. 1997. *Aging and assistive technology use and needs in adults with cerebral palsy living in community settings*. Chicago: Institute on Disability and Human Development, University of Illinois at Chicago.

Mendelson, L. S., Heller, T., and Factor, A. 1995. The transition from nursing homes to community living for people with developmental disabilities: An assessment of the assistive technology needs and usage. *Technology and Disability* 4:261–68.

Minihan, P., and Dean, D. 1990. Meeting the health services needs of persons with mental retardation living in the community. *American Journal of Public Health* 80:1043–48.

National Council on Disability. 1993. *Meeting the unique needs of minorities with disabilities: A report to the President and the Congress*. Washington, D.C.: National Council on Disability.

National Council on Disability. 1996. *Achieving independence: The challenge for the 21st century*. Washington, D.C.: National Council on Disability.

Pederson, E., and Nelis, T. 1997. Leadership partnership research and training for persons with mental retardation, their support people and other members of decision-making groups. Presentation at the International Roundtable on Aging and Intellectual Disability, Chicago.

Preston, L., and Heller, T. 1996. Working partnerships to individualize future planning for older families from diverse groups. Paper presented at the Sixth Lexington Conference on Aging and Developmental Disabilities, Lexington, Ky.

Prouty, R. W., and Lakin, K. C., eds. 1996. *Residential services for people with developmental disabilities: Status and trends through 1995.* Minneapolis: University of Minnesota, Research and Training Center on Community Living, Institute on Community Integration.

Rubin, S., Rimmer, J., Chicoine, B., Braddock, D., and McGuire, D. 1998. Overweight prevalence in persons with Down syndrome. *Mental Retardation* 36:175–81.

Stone, J. 1994. *Community living options: Family funded, individually owned, or shared.* Monograph 2. Lexington: University of Kentucky, Interdisciplinary Human Development Institute, Rehabilitation Research and Training Center on Aging with Mental Retardation.

Susa, C., and Clark, P. 1996. *Drafting a blueprint for change: The coordinator's manual.* Kingston: University of Rhode Island.

Sutton, E., Heller, T., Sterns, H., Factor, A., and Miklos, S. 1993. *Person-centered planning for later life: A curriculum for adults with mental retardation.* Akron: Rehabilitation Research and Training Center on Aging with Mental Retardation: University of Illinois at Chicago and the University of Akron.

Wehmeyer, M. L. 1995. The use of assistive technology by people with mental retardation and barriers to this outcome: A pilot study. *Technology and Disability* 4:195–204.

Yamaki, K., and Fujiura, G. 1999. *Employment and income status of adults with developmental disabilities living in the community.* Chicago: Department of Disability and Human Development, University of Illinois at Chicago.

Part 5

Future Directions

13

Methodological Issues

James S. Krause, Ph.D., and Rodney H. Adkins, Ph.D.

Underlying Principles

There are many reasons to investigate aging in the general population: investigations of health and health care needs are vital. These studies may address physical capacities, intellectual capacities, or social behaviors, patterns of activities, adaptations to retirement from employment, and reactions to the death of a spouse.

There are also many reasons to study aging associated with disability. First, while health, function, and emotional status change in the nondisabled population, given the nature and severity of issues facing people with disabilities, the magnitude and character of aging are likely to be different. Thus knowledge and policies based on studies of aging in the general population may not be entirely applicable to those with disabilities. Second, many government and private programs have been developed to help people with disabilities meet their needs in various aspects of their lives. If these programs are to be successful, they must be based on a comprehensive understanding of factors that affect the lives of people with disabilities. Aging is a special factor that requires particular investigation, since some programs may need to target individuals in a particular age group. Third, as individuals age with disabilities, their support systems also age. They may experience changes such as the death of a spouse or the loss of a primary caregiver. These types of losses may be critical to their lives, and during their lifetimes their support systems may go through several changes in both size and quality. These changes in, or losses of, tangible support (e.g., hands-on care) and intangible support (e.g., emotional sustenance) may in turn change the process of aging for those with disabilities. Fourth, their activity patterns may change more substantially with advancing age. For instance, some research has shown that individuals with spinal cord injury are more likely to leave the workforce prematurely (Krause 1992; Krause et al. 1998). Loss of gainful employment is associated with a decline in both tangible and intangible benefits, since both income and quality of life are compromised (Krause 1996; Krause and Anson 1997).

Underlying many of the aging changes experienced by those with and without disabilities are concomitant changes in health. While investigations of changes in health and health care needs are common in the general population, there is a large gap in knowledge comparing aging-related health changes in nondisabled and disabled people. For instance, studies are needed to determine whether the health of people with disabilities changes at the same rate as that of the general population or whether changes occur earlier among people with disabilities. It is also important to determine whether changes in health place individuals with disabilities at greater risk for adverse outcomes. For instance, long-term polio survivors are known to have a greater risk for diminished muscle function as they age (Halstead and Silver 2000). This "overuse syndrome" is thought to result from using some muscles to compensate for the loss of others (e.g., propelling a wheelchair rather than walking). In addition, particular types of medical problems may arise earlier or more often among people with disabilities, such as cardiovascular disease, diabetes, obesity, sleep apnea, digestive disorders, pulmonary and renal compromise, or certain neuromuscular conditions including osteoarthritis, osteoporosis, curvature the spine, chronic pain, and contractures (Charlifue, Weitzenkamp, and Whiteneck 1999). The net effect of aging may be increased disability, including loss of independence and diminished quality of life. A primary goal of these investigations must be to establish a basis for developing interventions and prevention strategies to treat conditions as they arise as well as to prevent them from occurring.

With regard to the latter, it is particularly important to recognize that the study of aging should not be restricted to aged people and that aging is a dynamic process. In the nondisabled population, aging is a gradual biological decline that begins as early as twenty-five years of age and accelerates more noticeably after the chronological age of forty to fifty (Charlifue, Weitzenkamp, and Whiteneck 1999). To approach the goal of fully understanding the aging process, we must examine the complete continuum, not just the far end (only older people). Among other problems, research that focuses on the far end of the continuum alone restricts knowledge of aging to the aged. While health care providers may observe certain problems only in elderly people, they may have had their genesis years or decades earlier. If the processes that led to these problems are not understood, we cannot prevent them in future elderly people.

From a methodological perspective, studies that concentrate only on aged people provide a biased depiction of aging, because only those who have survived to late life are represented. The further along on the age continuum research takes place, the more biased the image may be, because those on the far end may have an unusual advantage in one form or another. Their environment, which has influenced their life span, may have been less harsh than that of their peers; they may have been more adaptable; or their genetic structure may be more suited to a longer life. Nevertheless, those individuals who outlive most of their peers may be no more representative of individuals born at approximately the same time than are those in that group who died at a very early age. In situations where rapid and substantial advances have occurred, researchers must be cautious when comparing long-term survivors to younger groups. When we compare group averages, depending on the basis of comparison, long-term survivors can appear to have better outcomes, which can lead to an erroneous conclusion that people improve as they age. In reality, mortality after disability is a selective process whereby individuals who are in the best health and who are the best adjusted survive the longest (Krause et al. 1997; Krause 1999). This "survivor effect" occurs when selective attrition due to mortality makes it appear as though age is associated with positive changes in outcomes when in reality those who continue to survive are those who are best adjusted. When the focus of aging research is the aged, care must be taken to consider the findings from the perspective of this survival effect.

Aging and the Era Effect

In its simplest form, aging is the effect of the passage of time. Chronological age is an expression of the passage of time and is the component most commonly considered when researchers investigate the consequences of aging. However, the passage of a finite amount of time (e.g., fifty years) can occur anywhere along the infinite continuum of time. Thus people can age to the chronological age of fifty between the years 1900 and 1950, or between 1950 and 2000, or during any other fifty-year era. But the consequences of the passage of the fifty years during markedly different eras are likely to be different. Therefore the consequences observed as the effects of aging really consist of the effects of time expressed as chronological age plus the effects of the era when the passage of time took place. "Era effects" might be quite different for different outcomes. For example, during one era social conditions might be stable whereas scientific and medical fields might be advancing rapidly, which would result in minimal era effects for psychosocial outcomes but strong era effects for health outcomes. Imagine comparing aging effects just before the development of antibiotics with aging effects five or ten years after antibiotics were introduced.

In research jargon, era effects are called cohort effects, and in general research on aging they have been identified with the age-period-cohort problem (Schaie 1965). The problem for researchers (and those who might have reason to interpret research findings) is to sort out the effects of (chronological) age from the effects of birth cohort (or era of birth) and the period when the research was or is conducted. Why is it important to separate these effects? If the observed consequences are due to the passage of time only (i.e., true aging), there may be little that can be done to alter them. But if they result from exposure to a particular era, perhaps something can be (or has been) done that will change the future consequences.

Among people with disabilities, other components of aging may need to be investigated beyond chronological age and era. Some disabilities are present at birth; and where they are not, additional factors may influence aging. In addition to era of birth, era of treatment following onset of disability should be considered as an influence on aging in the disabled. Individuals experiencing the same treatment era would be referred to as an event cohort, similar to the concept of birth cohort for those born in the same era. Rapid advancements in treatment may produce quite different aging patterns in individuals born at approximately the same time and with ages at disability onset only a few years apart. In addition to treatment era, actual age at disability onset and duration of the disability, or the time lived since onset, may also influence aging.

Age at the onset of disability is important for several reasons. First, there may be wide variations in the age when the disability occurs. This may influence comparisons within, but especially across, disability conditions. Some disabling conditions typically occur at birth (cerebral palsy, spina bifida), whereas other conditions have late onset (e.g., Alzheimer disease). Yet other conditions have a fairly narrow range of onset or are more likely to occur in a certain age range. For instance, multiple sclerosis is likely to occur in the thirties or forties, whereas the likelihood of a stroke increases with age, and stroke occurs primarily after age sixty. Conditions due to injury, such as traumatic brain injury or spinal cord injury (SCI), are much more likely to occur among individuals in their late teens to early adulthood, but they may occur at any age.

In situations when age at onset is relatively homogeneous, occurring after physical maturation and before the period of rapid physical decline, it is less likely to affect most outcomes to any great extent. Nevertheless, age at injury, even when it is relatively homogeneous within a group, should not be ignored as a potential contributor to outcomes, perhaps more to psychosocial than to physical outcomes. Physically, most individuals have reached a plateau between eighteen and thirty-five years of age; however, many psychosocial changes occur between these ages (e.g., marriages/divorce, development and establishment of scholastic and career paths). The interruption of these events by a disabling condition during that age range may influence their outcomes extensively, depending on when it occurs.

Another example of the importance of analyzing age at disability is the implication of age at onset for quality of life. The length of time an individual has lived before the onset of the disability will affect the type and quality of life afterward. Those whose disability begins at birth will have no experience living without a disability and therefore no basis for comparison. This may influence their emotional adaptation, depending on their experiences growing up with the disability and the types of support they have had. Whereas emotional adaptation may be enhanced by never having faced the changes brought about by adult onset disability, social integration may be compromised by never having lived without a disabling condition. Children with disabling conditions are sometimes sent to special schools or otherwise isolated from nondisabled peers and may therefore be restricted from certain types of experiences. Conditions with variable onset, such as spinal cord injury, may present different challenges depending on the age at onset. It is widely accepted and substantiated through published literature that an earlier age at onset is associated with better outcomes, whereas studies of individuals who are disabled at older ages report greatly diminished quality of life (Castle 1994; Dijkers et al. 1995).

Age at injury should also be considered in terms of sampling distributions, especially when the outcome of interest is a developmental process for which the impact of the disability could be exaggerated. Bone loss is a physical example. Bone development is highly influenced by age, and disabilities that decrease mobility may alter that development (Riggs et al. 1981, 1982). When bone development is retarded, bone loss with age will begin at an altered baseline. Similarly, in people without physical disabilities natural bone loss tends to occur after age fifty (Riggs et al. 1981, 1982). When a physical disability occurs after fifty, the baseline from which any disability-related bone loss would begin is likely to be lower (Garland et al. 2001).

Similar factors are related to the number of years lived with a disability. Although chronological age and years since onset are identical for those whose disability occurs at birth, years lived after the onset of disability may vary greatly from chronological age among those who have adult-onset disabilities. The longer one lives after a disabling condition occurs, , the longer one has to adapt to the limitations it imposes. In this sense, a greater number of years lived after the onset of disability may substantially enhance adaptation and quality of life. However, years lived after the onset of disability may have an adverse effect on health, such as what has been observed with postpolio syndrome, where the cumulative impact of overuse of certain muscles becomes more apparent with age (Halstead and Silver 2000). In short, having lived a long time with a disability may exact a great toll on health. Individuals whose disability begins very late in life will have little time to adapt to it but will not experience the full effect of aging with a disability.

One additional note on the relation between chronological age, age at onset, and duration of disability is important. In mathematical or statistical terms, these three factors are linearly dependent. This means that the value of one can be derived from the values of the other two (i.e., an individual who is thirty-nine and has been disabled for twenty years was nineteen at the onset of disability). This may seem trivial, but it means that the influence of all three factors cannot be assessed statistically at the same time. Analytically, the three possible combinations of pairs of the three factors (age and duration, age and age at onset, and age at injury and duration) must be assessed separately to determine their relative influences on any given outcome or set of outcomes.

It is clear from this brief overview of aging factors that each of the potential components of aging will have an impact on an individual with a disability. The relationships are likely to be complex and therefore require substantial investigation. The effects may not be additive or may not equally affect all areas of life.

Research Designs to Examine the Effects of Aging

Several research designs may be used to study aging, both within the general population and after disability. These include the three traditional methods and the more sophisticated sequential designs. The three traditional types of research designs are cross-sectional design, in which measures from multiple cohorts are compared at a single point in time; longitudinal, in which measures from a single cohort are compared at two or more different times; and time-lagged, in which measures from different cohorts are compared at different times. Sequential designs combine two or more aspects of these three traditional designs in order to circumvent some of their limitations.

Traditional Designs

The cross-sectional design is the most commonly used method in aging studies, presumably because it is the quickest, easiest, and least expensive to employ. Using this design, outcomes are compared among either age or event cohorts (e.g., time since the onset of a disability). For example, age cohorts are commonly used to study such relationships as aging and IQ. Participants would be grouped according to age cohorts (e.g., five-year intervals: 21-25, 26-30, . . . 66-70) and IQ scores would be compared between cohorts, with any differences being interpreted as an aging effect. In studies of disability, outcomes—such as pain or urological function—might be compared between participants grouped into cohorts based on age (birth cohort), age at onset, or duration of disability. Any observed differences in outcomes would be attributed to aspects of aging. For example, one could randomly select samples of people with SCI who were twenty-five, thirty-five, or forty-five years old and measure severity of shoulder pain among all participants. One would then compare the mean pain severity scores of the three groups, with any statistically significant differences between cohorts attributed to aging.

A second aging factor applies to some people with disabilities—time since the onset of a disability (i.e., an event cohort). In some cases a researcher may be interested in aging after disability onset rather than aging per se. For example, a researcher may compare pain severity scores between cohorts of individuals who lived different lengths of time after a traumatic injury (e.g., 0-5 years, 6-10 years) to determine how aging after injury is associated with pain severity.

The major problem with the cross-sectional design is that the results are confounded with the cohorts. In the first example cited, age is confounded with birth cohort. Since people in the same birth cohort have experienced the same general environments over time (have lived in the same era), the observed differences in adjustment may reflect the effect of shared experiences among those in the oldest cohorts, such as living in an era when people with disabilities were viewed in a more negative light, rather than the effects of aging per se.

Cohort effects may also have an impact on people from event cohorts. For instance, the year or time period (e.g., decade) when disability began will be related to the types of rehabilitation programs and resources available during critical periods. With amputations, certain types of prostheses may have been available during one period but not earlier. With a spinal cord injury, length of rehabilitation stay and quality of care vary over time. Any observed differences in outcomes between cohorts based on time since disability onset may reflect differential access to resources owing to the timing of disability rather than the effects of time since onset per se. This is very important to consider, given the dramatic changes in rehabilitative programs in the managed care era.

In sum, although the cross-sectional design helps to describe the relation between age or time since disability onset and outcomes at a given point, it does not indicate how outcomes change over time or how environmental changes and era effects influence outcomes.

Using the longitudinal design, actual changes within individuals are measured over time. Therefore measurements are taken from a cohort on more than one occasion and the observations are compared across different points in time. For example, a researcher could randomly select a sample of participants without regard to age or time since disability onset and administer a pain severity measure on two or more occasions, separated by a significant interval (e.g., five years). Changes in pain severity scores between the two occasions would be attributed to aging.

Although the longitudinal design is generally accepted as the most appropriate for studying aging, it also has a major limitation in that it confounds aging with period (i.e., time of measurement). For example, if two administrations of an adjustment measure, in 1980 and 1990, showed that a group's pain severity scores declined over that period, this could be due to aging, or it could be the result of unique environmental changes that occurred during that decade (such as the development of a new intervention for pain). Examples of environmental changes may be changes in rehabilitation practices owing to reimbursement patterns within the insurance industry, the development of new technologies to assist people with disabilities, or the passing of legislation that either favorably or unfavorably affects outcomes. Similarly, other confounding factors, such as time since disability onset, may also contribute to the findings.

A practical limitation of the longitudinal design is the difficulty inherent in studying a group of participants over an extensive period. Attrition in longitudinal studies may occur for a number of reasons such as mortality, geographic mobility—inability to locate participants—and refusal to participate. Even when people are willing and able to respond, high mortality rates and geographic mobility may substantially reduce the overall response rate and compromise the validity of any given study.

In contrast to these other methods, the rarely used time-lagged design allows for investigating the impact of a changing environment by comparing measurements from one cohort at one point with those from a similar cohort taken at a later time. This design specifically addresses the association of era with outcomes by drawing samples that are intended to be equal in all respects other than the time when the measurements are taken. For example, the employment rate for individuals with a particular type of disabling condition could be calculated for one cohort in 1980 and compared with those from a different cohort in 1990. The cohorts would be matched on key characteristics such as age, gender, and time since disability onset, so that the samples would be taken from the same general population but at different times. Since the cohorts would comprise different individuals and no repeated measures would be taken (as with the longitudinal design), any observed differences between groups would be attributed to differences in the overall environment between the two times of measurement. Because independent samples are drawn at two different points, the time-lagged design isolates the effect of the environment from any changes due to aging. It therefore does not measure aging but aids in the interpretation of aging studies that use the cross-sectional and longitudinal methods by assessing era effects that are confounded in these designs. The primary limitations of the design are that the two samples must be drawn from the same population, and the design can identify only the influence of the general environmental change rather than the effects of specific components of the environment, such as a particular piece of legislation.

Table 13.1. Elements of the three basic research designs

	Cross-sectional	Longitudinal	Time-lagged
Number of cohorts	Multiple	Single	Single
Times of measurement	Single	Multiple	Multiple
Repeated measures (same participants)	No	Yes	No
Relevance to aging	Identifies differences between age cohorts	Identifies actual changes over time	Identifies changes of parallel cohorts to identify time changes

It is noteworthy that, under certain conditions, the longitudinal and time-lagged designs generate similar results. For example, in the case where an outcome is unrelated to aging but is influenced by environmental change, both designs will produce similar results by tapping the environmental effects. Similar results would also be obtained between longitudinal and time-lagged designs if aging affected an outcome but two components of aging (such as chronological age and time since disability onset) were each correlated with the outcome but in different directions (one positive, one negative). In these circumstances, the effects may balance out (table 13.1).

Alternative Designs

One means of eliminating some of the problems with the traditional designs is to incorporate into a single study components of multiple designs, such as cross-sequential and time-sequential. The cross-sequential design (Schaie 1965) combines aspects of both cross-sectional and longitudinal designs. A single cross-sectional sample is drawn, and observations are taken on two or more occasions. Longitudinal changes in adjustment are measured for each of the cohorts rather than for the sample as a whole (as is done with the traditional longitudinal design).

For example, scores for activities of daily living (ADLs) could be obtained from a cross-sectional sample in 1985 based on age (20–29, 40–49, 60–69) and again from the same sample in 1995. Comparing scores between the two times of measurement for each cohort would determine actual changes in ADLs over time within each cohort. If there were differences between cohorts in either the direction or the amount of change, then an interaction would be observed between the cohorts and time of measurement. By comparing the interaction between each age cohort at first testing (cross-sectional component) and change between the two times of measurement (longitudinal component), researchers can identify critical periods for change and obtain a true picture of aging. One possible interaction would be if ADL function does not change over time for people in the youngest age groups but declines for those in the oldest groups.

In sum, the cross-sequential design has the benefit of identifying actual longitudinal changes among the same individuals while circumventing the issues related to era effects before enrollment in the study (cross-sectional design limitation). The cross-sequential design is able to do this without the study of people over extensive periods as is necessary with the traditional longitudinal design. However, issues related to environmental or era effects between times of measurement remain confounded.

The time-sequential design also combines aspects of two traditional designs—cross-sectional and time-lagged (Schaie 1965). When using this design, two cross-sectional samples are drawn from the same population at two points in time. Cross-sectional comparisons are made by comparing outcomes between the cross-sectional cohorts, summing across the two times of measurement (i.e., combining the two samples). Time-lagged comparisons are made by comparing the responses between the two times of measurement, summing across the age cohorts (i.e., comparing the responses of the two samples). For example, one might obtain ADL scores from a sample of people from three age cohorts in 1985 (e.g., thirty, forty, and fifty years of age) and compare these scores with those from a different sample divided into the same age groupings in 1995. Comparing differences in the scores between the two times of measurement (between the two samples) would tap the effects of environmental change or era effects between the two times of measurement (time-lagged analysis). Time-sequential designs have been used to identify the role of the environment in adjustment after SCI (Krause and Crewe 1991; Krause and Sternberg, 1997; see table 13.2).

Measurement Issues

To adequately address research issues of aging with disabilities, one must understand some aspects of longitudinal measurement. Beyond the problems of

Table 13.2. Comparison of sequential and basic research designs

	Cross-sequential	Time-sequential
Cross-sectional	Yes	Yes
Longitudinal	Yes	No
Time-lagged	No	Yes
Advantages	Identifies longitudinal (repeated measures) changes related to aging while identifying these effects for different cohorts	Assesses the effects of period between times of measurement while identifying these effects for different cohorts

period of measurement, era and survival effects, and participant attrition, the measures used must also be of concern. Just as treatment progresses, so do measurement tools. New measures and measurement techniques are constantly being developed and old/obsolete/inadequate ones are constantly being replaced. This applies to tools for physical measurement as well as paper and pencil measures, such as the continual development of more sophisticated radiological techniques (i.e., from simple x-ray to CT scans to MRI). This turnover of measurement methods and tools can be a disadvantage for research, especially long-term longitudinal research. Measurement methods and tools used in the initial phases of a longitudinal project may be considered inappropriate or obsolete or, worse, may be unavailable during later phases of a multiple-year project. And though newer and perhaps better measurement tools may become available, it is impossible to return to the past and obtain new measures. When this occurs, there is always the temptation to continue to collect data with the initial tools, if possible, and to add the new ones. However, this can drain resources and lead to an unwieldy or infeasible project with no usable results. From this perspective, including only the most stable measures should be considered before embarking on a longitudinal project, especially one intended to be long-term.

Several measurement issues are not specific to the study of either aging or disability but are general scientific principles that are addressed in all similar types of research. Two primary issues include the level of measurement of the variable and the psychometric properties of the measuring instrument. Level of measurement refers to the types of data being collected (e.g., gender, height, weight). Psychometric properties reflect the quality of specific measurement instruments that are used to measure variables such as subjective strength, function, or pain, or psychological variables such as depression.

Level of Measurement

There are four levels of measurement: nominal, ordinal, interval, and ratio. The level of measurement used has implications for the types of data being collected and the types of statistical analyses that can therefore be performed.

Nominal data are categorical in nature (they cannot be quantified). Gender is an example of nominal data. Simple counts and percentages are the only types of statistical descriptions that can be performed on nominal variables (e.g., there were seven women and thirteen men; 35 percent were women). Categorical variables may also be cross-tabulated. For instance, in addition to reporting a percentage of a sample with one characteristic, such as 35 percent were women, percentage can be calculated on two or more characteristics (e.g., 20 percent were Caucasian women).

Ordinal measurement is not strictly categorical in nature, since it implies that the variable can be quantified in such a way that one variable has more or less of some quality than another variable. Examples of ordinal measurement include rank orders. For instance, a physical or occupational therapist may be asked to rank three individuals on how well they performed a certain activity, such as dressing, with the individual who performed best ranked as 1, the second as 2, and the third as 3. The rank order of the individuals may be compared between raters to determine whether different people tended to use the same rank ordering (ranked the individuals in the same order). However, there is no assumption that the intervals between the ranks are equal. In this example, you would not be able to conclude that the difference between the individuals who were ranked as 1 and 2 was equal to the interval between those ranked 2 and 3. For instance, the person whose performance ranked second may have performed nearly as well as the person whose performance was ranked as the best, whereas the person ranked third may not have performed well at all. Statistics that use rank order, such as the Spearman rank order correlation, are appropriate with ordinal measurement. They may provide an index of association between independent rankings by different individuals.

Interval measurement represents a substantial improvement over nominal or ordinal measurement. With interval measurement, the difference in magnitude between two numbers may be compared. Again using the example of dressing, suppose individuals were asked to rate performance on a scale of 1 to 5, with 1 being poor and 5 being excellent. You can obtain an average performance for the three ratings. Assume that several judges rated the performance of three individuals and the average for individual 1 was 5.0, the average for individual 2 was 4.0, and the average for individual 3 was only 2.0. Because the measurement is interval, you can say that the interval between individuals 1 and 2 was half that of the interval between individuals 2 and 3 (making assumptions regarding the scaling). However, with interval measurement there is no true zero point.

The last type of measurement is ratio, which is identical to interval measurement with the added enhancement that it has a true zero point. Weight is a ratio measurement because there is a real zero weight. In the previous example, ratio data would be used if performance were measured in time to complete the task. All statistical methods may be used with ratio scales. However, in reality, ratio characteristics are generally assumed when applying statistical methods to interval data. In data analysis, this has generally become the common practice.

Psychometric Properties

Many variables that are the focus of investigation in the social and behavioral sciences require the development of special measurement instruments. The constructs that are measured are generally theoretical in nature, making measurement complex. For contrast, in the physical sciences, measuring variables such as height is straightforward, since there is no disagreement as to what constitutes height (although the units of measure may be open to debate—inches versus centimeters). However, constructs such as "adjustment to disability" are theoretical, since they assume an underlying construct. Different researchers may disagree on what elements constitute adjustment, or whether adjustment is a unidimensional or multidimensional construct (one score versus multiple scores). The goal of measurement is to produce instruments that measure a construct, such as adjustment, in both a reliable and a valid fashion, so that researchers at different locations may administer the same instrument and interpret the scores in similar fashion.

Two basic types of data are collected with regard to any particular instrument: reliability and validity. Reliability refers to whether the measurement instrument will consistently produce the same or similar scores across different locations, testers, subtests, or general circumstances. Reliability does not imply that the instrument measures the intended construct.

Several types of reliability may be collected on a given instrument. The most commonly used indicator is internal consistency. This refers to the extent to which the items are internally consistent or measure a similar construct. Internal consistency reliability is calculated by computing correlation coefficients (or the association) between items that are used to measure a single construct. For instance, the items that constitute an adjustment measure should be highly correlated if they indeed measure the same construct. Therefore we would anticipate that individuals who respond positively to one item indicating that they are well adjusted would respond positively to similar items (again indicating that they are well adjusted). If a scale is not internally consistent, then the instrument would have poor reliability. If a particular instrument contains more than one scale, each scale should have high internal consistency reliability (the items within that scale should be highly correlated).

A second measure of reliability is split-half reliability. Rather than computing the intercorrelations of all scale items, split-half reliability correlates scores on half the items with scores on the other half. If the scale is reliable, individuals who score high on one half of the items should also score high on the other half.

A third type of reliability is alternative forms. This type of reliability can be calculated if there is more than one form of the instrument. Administering both forms to a group of participants allows one to correlate the scores on both forms with each other. As with other types of reliability, individuals who score high on one form should also score high on the alternative form.

A fourth indicator of reliability is different in its nature from those just described. To determine test-retest reliability, the measurement instrument is administered to the same group of individuals on two occasions and the scores are correlated between the two occasions. Provided the construct itself is not changed substantially over time and that the interval between measurements is relatively short, then individuals who score high on one occasion should also score high on the second occasion. Test-retest is generally the most stringent test of reliability.

Validity

In addition to determining whether a measuring instrument is internally consistent and produces consistent measurements across time (reliability), it is important to determine whether it measures what it intends to measure (whether it is valid). Validity is the ultimate test, then, in instrument utility.

There are several types of validity. Face validity refers how well the questions appear to measure the intended construct. For instance, a measure of adjustment to disability would have face validity if it asked people how they were adjusting. In reality, face validity is not a measure of validity in the psychometric sense, since no psychometric data are collected. Yet it often helps to establish rapport with the person who is completing the questionnaire.

Content validity refers to how adequately the instrument taps the entire content domain. Again with regard to the example of a measure of adjustment to disability, content validity would be achieved if the measure adequately sampled the full domain of aspects of adjustment rather than only selective aspects.

The most important kind of validity is construct validity. In essence, all types of validity are forms of construct validity. Construct validity is how well the instrument truly measures the theoretical construct of interest. In the previous example, a measure of adjustment should measure how successfully individuals adapt to disability rather than whether they are depressed or exhibiting another form of psychopathology. There are two key components to construct validity: convergent validity and discriminant validity. Convergent validity occurs when independent measures of a single construct obtained through different methods are highly correlated. For instance, a self-report measure of depression would show convergent validity if it was highly correlated with biological or observational measures of depression. In contrast, discriminant validity occurs when two distinct constructs are measured using similar methods but the correlation between measures is low. If individuals completed self-report measures of depression and sensation seeking, divergent validity would occur if the two measures were minimally correlated despite using similar methods of measurement. It is important to demonstrate discriminant validity to show that method variance (using the same data collection method) does not account for any observed correlation between measures, as would be the case if two measures of the same construct, both using the same method, were correlated (e.g., two self-report measures of depression). In sum, construct validity occurs when independent measures of a single construct are correlated with each other (convergent validity), but are not highly correlated with measures of other constructs using the same method (divergent validity).

Statistical Methods

Although daunting to students and many researchers, statistical methods are perhaps the most valuable tool available to aging and disability investigators. The sophisticated research designs described earlier (cross-sequential, time-sequential) would have little meaning were it not for the availability of appropriate statistical methods with which to analyze and interpret the data. The study of aging is enhanced by certain types of statistical methods, particularly those that allow age effects to be partitioned (different components of aging may be investigated simultaneously). In addition, certain types of trend analysis help us understand the shape of the relation between aging and outcomes, since this relation is not only linear. For instance, declines in physical functioning with age may not follow a linear pattern; function may remain stable for long periods, with rapid declines observed at a given time.

There are two primary types of statistical analysis: descriptive and inferential. Descriptive statistics are the most basic type of data analytic methods. They are used simply to describe a group of observations, such as the age of a particular group of people. There is no attempt to draw inferences about a larger population but only to describe the observations at hand. The most common descriptive statistics relate to central tendency and to the spread or dispersion of observations. The three types of central tendency are the mean (mathematical average), the median (the middle observation when scores are ranged from lowest to highest), and the mode (the most frequent observation). For example, if there were five individuals whose ages were 10, 10, 15, 20, and 35, the mode would be 10, the median would be 15, and the average (or mean) would be 18.

Measures of dispersion are somewhat more complex. Measures of central tendency include the standard deviation and the range. The standard deviation is a statistic that measures dispersion around the mean and is calculated by taking the square root of the sum of each observation's squared deviation from the mean, divided by the number of observations. It is generally used when the mean is the measure of central tendency. The range or a special case of the range (interquartile range) is used when the median is the measure of central tendency. It is beyond the scope of this chapter to detail formulas for these measures, yet it is important to understand that researchers must measure both central tendency and dispersion to adequately describe their observations. For instance, if the average income of people working at a particular company was $25,000 per year (the indicator of central tendency) and the salaries ranged from $15,000 to $35,000 per year, there would be a relatively narrow range of salaries. The situation would be quite different if the average salary was $25,000 but the range was $10,000 to $100,000.

Several other types of descriptive statistics are used to show the distribution of observations. A normal distribution occurs when the mean, mode, and median are the same value and observations are equally distributed through the tails of the distribution. A normal distribution is often referred to as a bell-shaped curve. The example of salaries where the average was $25,000 and the range was $15,000 to $35,000 would approximate a normal distribution (more information would be needed to determine whether it fully fit that pattern). However, the case where the average salary was $25,000, the lowest salary was $10,000, and the highest salary was $100,000 clearly is not a normal distribution. Where there are extreme observations, these outlying scores will have a dramatic impact on the mean, but not on the median. In these cases the median will have a score lower than the mean and will be a more informative and less volatile measure of central tendency.

Another descriptive statistic is the correlation coefficient, an index of the association between two sets of observations. Correlation coefficients range from 0 to 1 (-1.00 to 1.00), with 0 indicating no association and 1.00 indicating a perfect correlation. A correlation exists when scores on one variable are associated with scores on another variable. For instance, height and weight are correlated. Across a group of people, those who are taller will tend to weigh more. However, the correlation will be far from perfect, since there will be some people who are underweight for their height and others who are overweight for their height. Another example is pay scale, where there is generally a correlation between years worked at a particular job and income because raises are at least partially determined by tenure. If a rigid pay scale was in place with a specified starting rate that increased only by years on the job, the correlation would be perfect (1.00), since employees' pay would simply reflect their tenure. If other factors were considered, such as performance, then the correlation would be less than 1.00.

Note that correlation coefficients may be positive or negative. An example of a negative correlation would be the relation between smoking and life expectancy, since the greater the number of cigarettes smoked, the lower the life expectancy. The magnitude of the correlation is not determined by whether the correlation is positive or negative, since a correlation of $-.78$ is greater than the correlations of $-.22$, $+.08$, or $+.67$. Also note that a correlation between two variables does not imply causation. A significant correlation between two variables may be completely causative (the rigid pay scale example), partially causative (smoking is one variable contributing to diminished life expectancy), or not causative at all.

Inferential statistics are much more important to researchers than descriptive statistics. Whereas descriptive statistics are used to summarize a specific set of observations, inferential statistics are used to form conclusions about observations taken from a sample drawn from a larger population in order to make conclusions about the larger population. Tests of statistical significance are fundamental to inferential statistics and involve testing specific hypotheses.

The differences between descriptive and inferential statistics are clarified in the following example. A rehabilitation professional observes that people attending her clinic who used a particular type of wheelchair cushion (cushion A) seem to have had fewer pressure ulcers in the previous year than those who used a different cushion (cushion B). She therefore documents the number of pressure ulcers among the former patients, compares the average number of pressure ulcers between the two groups, and indeed finds that those with cushion A reported fewer pressure ulcers than those using cushion B. Because she was interested only in pressure ulcers of those particular former patients at that hospital and collected information only on those patients (i.e., the population of patients at that clinic), she is then able to conclude that, at this clinic, patients who used cushion A had fewer pressure ulcers than those using cushion B. She does not need inferential statistics to draw her conclusions.

Now suppose her interests change and she now wants to draw conclusions about differences between cushion A and cushion B within a larger population, say, either future patients at her clinic or patients in the entire country. Since she cannot collect data on all the patients in the country, she must use inferential statistics. To do so, she must first draw samples of individuals who use cushion A or cushion B from the larger population, collect data on their pressure ulcers, and then compare the mean numbers of pressure ulcers for the two groups. Unlike the example where she was interested only in pressure ulcers at her clinic and was able to use all observations, chance findings may occur when sampling from a larger population by virtue of the particular cases that are randomly selected. The researcher may have selected a sample of individuals with either very high or very low numbers of pressure ulcers simply by chance. She wants to know with some level of confidence that this has not occurred. Inferential statistics may be used to assess the probability that any observed differences between groups of observations occurred solely by chance.

Hypothesis testing is fundamental to inferential statistics. If the researcher wants to test the hypothesis that for a population of wheelchair users, those who use cushion A will have fewer pressure ulcers than those who use cushion B, she would first state the null hypothesis and then draw a sample of observations from each group. The null hypothesis states that there are no differences in pressure ulcers between the groups using the two cushions. The researcher's true interest is to reject the null hypothesis and accept an alternative hypothesis that the means are different. She will perform a test of statistical significance that compares the two means and computes the probability that the observed difference between them was likely to occur by chance.

Three parameters are central to significance testing: the magnitude of the differences between observations (in this case the difference between the two means); the variance of the observations (i.e., the degree of differences within each set of measures); and sample size. The larger the difference between the two means, the less likely that the difference is a function of chance. Whereas the mean is the measure of central tendency, the measure of dispersion is used to meaningfully evaluate the magnitude of the mean differences. For instance, a mean difference in pressure ulcers of two per year would be more meaningful if the average number of pressure ulcers was only one per year as opposed to five per year. The effect size is determined by dividing the difference between the two means by the standard deviation of observations—the square root of the variance. It is very important to consider effect size when drawing conclusions regarding the practical significance of a particular difference in means.

The additional parameter that must be considered with hypothesis testing is the size of the sample drawn from the population. Sample size is directly taken into account in the statistical analysis, and the larger the sample size, the greater the likelihood of obtaining statistically significant differences for any given effect size. This makes sense intuitively, since the larger the sample size selected, the less likely that random factors related to sampling could account for observed differences in means. For instance, if the average number of pressure ulcers was two per year in the population and only five cases were randomly selected, one of whom had had ten pressure ulcers in the past year, this individual will have a substantial effect on the mean, which may lead to erroneous conclusions when comparing two means. On the other hand, if fifty cases were selected, then, all things being equal, one person with ten pressure ulcers would not have a substantial effect on the mean.

The accepted probability for rejecting the null hypothesis that two means are equal is .05 (one in twenty or less). This means that to have scientific credibility, there must be no more than a 5 percent likelihood that these observed differences occurred by chance. In some cases, a more stringent criterion will be used to determine statistical significance. This typically depends on the importance of the findings and the researcher's desire to avoid concluding that differences exist when, in reality, there are no differences in the populations.

Statistical significance should not be confused with practical or clinical significance. Very small differences may be statistically significant if the sample size used in a particular study is exceedingly large. A large sample size increases the researcher's power to identify a truly significant difference between two sets of observations. However, effect size is of greater clinical or practical significance. As stated earlier, effect size refers to the difference in magnitude between two sets of observations divided by the standard deviation of the observations. It does not take into account the sample size or number of observations.

For instance, based on the previous example, a researcher may want to see if changing from cushion B to cushion A reduces the number of pressure ulcers observed over the next year. Therefore she randomly divides the users of wheelchair cushion B into two groups—those who continue using cushion B and those who switch to cushion A—and then counts the number of pressure ulcers in each group over the next year. Assume that the number of pressure ulcers drops by half among those who switched to cushion A, whereas no changes are observed in pressure ulcers among those who continue using cushion B. This magnitude of change would indicate a clinically significant or relevant decrease in pressure ulcers and would have a rather large effect size given the magnitude of change associated with the intervention. But the difference may not be statistically significant if there were only five individuals in each group. If the sample size in each group is increased, the likelihood that the finding is statistically significant increases, even if the effect size stays the same (i.e., pressure ulcers are reduced by 50 percent after switching cushions). Conversely, if the number of pressure ulcers declined by only 5 percent, this difference would not be clinically significant. However, if there were enough cases in each group—several hundred, for example—the findings may be statistically significant in that they were unlikely to occur by chance.

In sum, it is possible to have a statistically significant difference that is not particularly meaningful clinically; or there may be a clinically meaningful difference that is not statistically significant because a researcher has not invested enough resources to have the power (owing to small sample size) to detect a statistically significant difference.

Investigations of aging are complicated by the many methodological factors described throughout this chapter. One tool that is helpful in identifying the relation between aging and any given outcome is trend analysis. Correlation coefficients measure the linear association between two variables. Therefore they will detect associations between aging parameters and any given outcome as long as the relation is linear. In the real world, however, relations between aging variables and outcomes are often more complex. Curvilinear relations may also be observed between age and any given outcome. Certain health variables follow this pattern. Although not frequently observed in a given portion of the age range, such as investigations of adults, some characteristics may increase at one point on the aging parameter and decrease at the later point. Although these complex relations challenge to the researcher, trend analysis is a valuable tool to help us understand them. Given appropriate study designs, researchers can investigate these complex relations with the comfort of knowing that the statistical methods available to them are fully equipped to handle the complexities of aging.

Special Measurement Issues Related to Disability and Aging

Investigating outcomes after the onset of a disabling condition requires some conceptual clarity regarding terminology. There are three key terms: impairment, disability, and participation (formerly referred to as handicap). The World Health Organization has promoted a classification scheme using these three concepts. Impairment refers to the medical condition itself, such as a spinal cord injury or traumatic brain injury. Diagnostic categories are often used to describe impairment, such as the ASIA Motor Index for spinal cord injury that classifies individuals' injuries based on the combination of level and completeness of the injury. In contrast to the measurement of impairment, the measurement of disability focuses on functional limitations. The Functional Independence Measure (FIM) is the most widely used measure of independence with activities of daily living. The term "handicap" was generally restricted to an individual's ability to function within the community. However, the term "participation" has replaced "handicap." The Craig Handicap Assessment and Reporting Technique (CHART) (Whiteneck et al. 1992) was developed to measure handicap or participation in community settings, as was the Community Integration Questionnaire (CIQ) (Willer, Ottenbacher, and Coad 1994).

Impairment or diagnostic category is unlikely to change with age, but functional limitations (disability) may change with the natural decline in physical function associated with aging. Therefore individuals with a particular impairment such as polio may find it harder to perform self-care as they age. This may be a direct result of aging, or it may be related to the onset of other secondary conditions, also referred to as secondary disabilities. Participation or handicap also may change dramatically with age, as people may retire early from gainful employment, visit community settings less frequently, and otherwise change their patterns of activities as a result of both the disability and age.

Summary

Investigators who want to research aging after the onset of a disability face many challenges, but they also have great opportunities. We hope that in reading this chapter novice researchers in the field of aging with a disability are intrigued and enticed by the opportunity to investigate the basic human phenomenon of aging among special population(s) that may derive great benefit from their research. We also hope that new researchers will take comfort in learning that, while complex, the methodological tools are available to perform the needed studies.

As in all scientific endeavors, researchers who share a commitment to a particular area of investigation must be willing to develop an understanding of the necessary tools for their field of study. We hope that the readers of this chapter embrace the methodology that is available and enhance their commitment to the field of rehabilitation and disability by initiating needed studies of aging and disability. The ultimate benefits will be bestowed on those whose lives will be enhanced by diligent researchers who have focused their skill and effort on helping us to understand the impact of aging with a disability.

REFERENCES

Castle, R. 1994. An investigation into the employment and occupation of patients with a spinal cord injury. *Paraplegia* 32:182–87.

Charlifue, S. W., Weitzenkamp, D. A., and Whiteneck, G. G. 1999. Longitudinal outcomes in spinal cord injury: Aging, secondary conditions, and well-being. *Archives of Physical Medicine and Rehabilitation* 80:1429–34.

Dijkers, M. P., Abela, M. B., Gans, B. M., and Gordon, W. A. 1995. The aftermath of spinal cord injury. In *Spinal cord injury: Clinical outcomes from the model systems*, ed. S. L. Stover, J. A. DeLisa, and G. G. Whiteneck. Gaithersburg, Md.: Aspen.

Garland, D. E., Adkins, R. H., Rah, A., and Stewart, C. A. 2001. Bone loss with aging and the impact of SCI. *Topics in Spinal Cord Injury Rehabilitation* 6:47–60.

Halstead, L. S., and Silver, J. K. 2000. Non-paralytic polio and post-polio syndrome. *American Journal of Physical Medicine and Rehabilitation* 79:13–18.

Krause, J. S. 1992. Employment after spinal cord injury. *Archives of Physical Medicine and Rehabilitation* 73:163–69.

Krause, J. S. 1996. Employment after spinal cord injury: Transition and life adjustment. *Rehabilitation Counseling Bulletin* 39:244–55.

Krause, J. S. 1999. Measuring quality of life and secondary conditions: Experiences with spinal cord injury. In *Issues in disability and health: The role of secondary conditions and quality of life*, ed. R. Simeonsson and L. McDevitt. Chapel Hill: University of North Carolina, FPG Child Development Center.

Krause, J. S., and Anson, C. A. 1997. Adjustment after spinal cord injury: Relationship to participation in employment or educational activities. *Rehabilitation Counseling Bulletin* 40:202–14.

Krause, J. S., and Crewe, N. M. 1991. Chronologic age, time since injury, and time of measurement: Effect on adjustment after spinal cord injury. *Archives of Physical Medicine and Rehabilitation* 71:91–100.

Krause, J. S., and Sternberg, M. 1997. Aging and spinal cord injury: The role of chronologic age, time since injury and environmental change. *Rehabilitation Psychology* 42:287–302.

Krause, J. S., Sternberg, M., Maides, J., and Lottes, S. 1997. Mortality after spinal cord injury: An 11-year prospective study. *Archives of Physical Medicine and Rehabilitation* 78:815–21.

Krause, J. S., Sternberg, M., Maides, J., and Lottes, S. 1998. Employment after spinal cord injury: Differences related to geographic region, gender, and race. *Archives of Physical Medicine and Rehabilitation* 79:615–24.

Riggs, B. L., Whaner, H. W., Dunn, W. L., Mazess, R. B., Offord, K. P., and Melton, L. J., III. 1981. Differential changes in bone mineral density of the appendicular and axial skeleton with aging: Relationship to spinal osteoporosis. *Journal of Clinical Investigation* 67:328–35.

Riggs, B. L., Whaner, H. W., Seeman, E., Offord, K. P., Dunn, W. L., Mazess, R. B., Johnson, K. A., and Milton, L. J., III. 1982. Changes in bone mineral density of the proximal femur and spine with aging: Differences between the postmenopausal and senile osteoporosis syndromes. *Journal of Clinical Investigation* 70:716–23.

Schaie, W. K. 1965. A general model for the study of developmental problems. *Psychological Bulletin* 64:261–70.

Whiteneck, G. G., Charlifue, S. W., Gerhart, K. A., Overholser, J. D., and Richardson, G. N. 1992. Quantifying handicap: A new measure of long-term rehabilitation outcomes. *Archives of Physical Medicine and Rehabilitation* 73:519–26.

Willer, B., Ottenbacher, K. J., and Coad, M. L. 1994. The community integration questionnaire: A comparative examination. *American Journal of Physical Medicine and Rehabilitation* 73:103–11.

14

The Politics of Aging with a Disability

Health Care Policy and the Shaping of a Public Agenda

Fernando Torres-Gil, Ph.D., and Michelle Putnam, Ph.D.

The concerns of older people and people with disabilities have risen on the nation's political agenda. This political elevation reflects decades of advocacy, lobbying, and public awareness of people with social, economic, health, and physical vulnerabilities. Debates about entitlement programs such as Medicare and Medicaid illustrate the growing public awareness of those important issues. But the real test of how this country responds to the needs of people with disabilities will occur as two important demographic trends come to fruition: the aging of the Baby Boom population and the aging of people with long-term disabilities such as cerebral palsy, spinal cord injury, polio, and multiple sclerosis. Public policy actions, especially in the health area, will have major repercussions for both of these populations. Thus it becomes important for aging interest groups, disability organizations, and people of all ages with disabilities to pay close attention to political decisions and public policy actions over the next several years. Such actions will largely determine the extent of public benefits and services and possibly quality of life for people aging with disabilities.

This chapter assesses the interrelation of health policy and aging with a disability. It will present demographic data, discuss the importance of inter-est-group politics, examine the nature of health policy developments, raise is-

sues and concerns that people aging with disabilities may face as the population ages, emphasize the need to monitor the political process, and suggest
areas of action and advocacy. We assume that people with disabling conditions, particularly those now in midlife, have a major stake in public policy
decisions affecting health and long-term care programs such as Medicare
and Medicaid. Future political actions in these arenas will determine
whether people aging with disabilities will receive adequate health care in
old age.

The Demographic Imperative

The population of the United States is aging; this much is well known. The
2000 data from the Census Bureau reinforce the public recognition that the
number of older people is growing and longevity is increasing. The median
age in the United States increased from 32.9 years in 1990 to 35.3 in 2000 and
is expected to increase to thirty-nine or older by 2030 (U.S. Bureau of the
Census 1990, 1996, 2000). Since 1900, life expectancy has increased by
thirty-one years for women (from forty-eight to seventy-nine) and by
twenty-eight years for men (from forty-six to seventy-four). In the past century,
while the total U.S. population tripled (including those under sixty-five years
of age), the elderly population increased elevenfold (U.S. Bureau of the Census 1996). The elderly population is expected to grow substantially between
2010 and 2030 (U.S. Bureau of the Census 1996). While Census 2000 found
that 12.4 percent of the population is over sixty-five, that proportion is expected to increase to 15.7 percent by 2020 and to 21 percent by 2040 (Day
1993; U.S. Bureau of the Census 1996, 2000). By 2010, Baby Boomers will be
reaching retirement age; and when they become senior citizens (assuming we
continue to use current definitions of old age), the population of older people
will double to about 75 million.

People with severe disabilities are also enjoying increased longevity. Advances in technology, medicine, public health, and consumer awareness
have enabled those aging with long-term disabilities such as cerebral palsy,
polio, and spinal cord injuries—who in earlier times were not expected to
survive even into middle age—to move into old age. There are an estimated
600,000 to one million people living with polio, more than half of whom are
now fifty-five and older (Tompkins 1997). People with spinal cord injuries
are estimated to have a life expectancy that is 85 percent of that of the

nondisabled population (Sasma, Patrick, and Feusser 1993). According to Campbell, Sheets, and Strong (1999), gains in longevity are also occurring for people aging into disability (e.g., rheumatoid arthritis, stroke) for the first time in midlife to later life. They indicate, however, that there is a downside to increased longevity for people aging with disabilities and for those experiencing disabilities in midlife to later life. Many who have survived chronic physical disabilities experience new health problems and functional changes. For example, by age forty to fifty polio survivors face the recurring challenge of postpolio syndrome, including new fatigue, pain, muscle weakness, and greater limitations on mobility. Further, they say, "These later-life effects of primary disability are typically unanticipated by both consumers and providers and have the potential to further erode independence and reduce quality of life" (106). In an extensive review of the literature, Campbell, Sheets, and Strong (1999) found that most of the secondary conditions affecting those aging with disabilities were related to overuse of a weakened neuromuscular system; underuse or misuse of the neuromuscular system owing to gait problems and immobility or deconditioning; complications resulting from the original injury or disease or from the treatment and care received; poor lifestyle behaviors and coping strategies; and "environmental and attitudinal barriers on the part of society and/or the individual that limit access to preventive services and to opportunities for social promotion and health-promoting activities" (197). It is this last factor that concerns us here: To what extent can environmental and attitudinal barriers be overcome through public policy, and how much do interest group politics between organized groups for the disabled and older people hinder or enhance their effectiveness? These questions highlight the growing number of people with chronic conditions who will have an increased stake in political decisions regarding expanding public financing and public programs for people with disabilities, older people, and those aging with disabilities. According to a 1995 report on chronic care in America, an estimated 99 million people in the United States suffered from chronic conditions characterized by persistent and recurring health consequences lasting for some years (Robert Wood Johnson Foundation 1996). Of these, 28 million (28 percent) were limited in major activities. The number of people with chronic conditions will increase by approximately 35 million, resulting in 134 million people with chronic conditions.

Figure 14.1 shows that one in five disabled people today, a large percentage

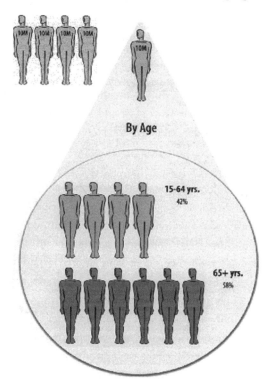

Figure 14.1. One in five disabled people needs help with basic activities of daily living. *Source:* J. M. McNeil, "Americans with Disabilities, 1991–92," U.S. Bureau of the Census. Data from the Survey of Income and Program Participation, 70–33. U.S. Bureau of the Census (1993), 9. *Note:* Population consists of those fifteen and older living in the community. This estimate of the number of disabled persons includes both those with activity limitations and those needing help with activities of daily living (ADLs) or instrumental activities of daily living (IADLs). Activity limitation means a long-term reduction in the capacity to perform the average kind or amount of activities appropriate to one's age group (e.g., going to school, going to work, living independently). ADLs include bathing, dressing, eating, walking, and other personal care. IADLs include preparing meals, shopping, using the telephone, managing money, taking medications, doing light housework, and other measures of living independently.

of whom are under sixty-five, need help with basic daily activities. If current trends continue, most of these people will be living longer than their counterparts in the past. Thus people with disabilities will find that issues of aging, old-age politics, and public policy debates about health care and long-term care programs for aging populations are becoming relevant to them.

Generational Politics

One key element in understanding the demographic imperative is the concept of generational politics and cohort analysis. Generational cohorts are distinct populations of individuals, born during the same periods, who are aging with similar historical experiences (Torres-Gil and Villa 2000). Today's cohort of people aged seventy and older, known as the New Deal cohort, was raised during the Depression, World War II, and the accompanying Cold War. The post–World War II generation, known as the Baby Boomer cohort, grew up in an era of civil rights, tolerance, prosperity, and civic activism. Baby Boomers grew up in an era of the Great Society and during a period of civil rights agitation. Future cohorts, today's younger Generation X (those now in their twenties and thirties) and the Baby Boomlet (kindergarten through grade twelve and college age) have their own set of generational experiences, especially those involving the advent of the information age. Each cohort views its needs and its own aging differently, and they may have differing views on the role of government and public policy. In the current landscape of generational politics, the New Deal cohort appears to be most supportive of preserving the current arrangement of age-based, categorical entitlement programs such as Social Security and Medicare. And early indications are that the Generation X cohort will support privatizing entitlement programs, in part because of doubts about Social Security's solvency. These differences in how generations view aging will influence the public policy debates about the types of safety nets and public benefits that should be available to older adults and must be factored into the analysis of interest-group politics. For example, the most prominent senior citizen advocates are from the New Deal cohort, while many disability activists are Baby Boomers. How senior citizens and disability activists address their cohort issues may influence their ability to establish coalitions.

Interest-group politics refers to individuals and groups organizing, advocating, and lobbying for their particular interests. The nature of American democracy gives great credence to organized groups and provides many opportunities to influence Congress and state legislatures, the courts, federal and state bureaucracies, and public opinion. Thus, how well such groups can articulate their position, promote their case, and influence political decision makers will significantly determine their success in shaping public policy. The ability of people with long-term disabilities to organize and to influence public policies affecting their concerns will be more and more important in the next few years as major debates about Medicare and Medicaid unfold. The political decisions made during this time will shape the levels and types of benefits and eligibility for these programs as well as their provisions, including prescription drugs, home- and community-based services, and access to technology.

Over the past half century, older people have become particularly effective at interest-group politics and are considered an important political lobby (Torres-Gil 1992). Their long-term efforts to influence public policy, beginning during the Great Depression, have left an indelible mark on the political landscape and created the "politics of aging." In part this is because older people vote more often than other age groups; they are well-organized at the national, state, and local levels; and they enjoy a high level of political credibility (Day 1990). Aging interest groups range from the Older Women's League to the National Committee to Preserve Social Security and Medicare to AARP (formerly the American Association of Retired Persons). The aging lobby may not always be successful in seeking redress from Congress or state legislatures, but its members are always heard and can shape the nature of political debates, particularly around entitlement programs.

People with disabilities, on the other hand, have limited experience in operating within the politics of aging. The focus of disability activism has historically been on education, rehabilitation, independent living, and work-related policy. Although health and long-term care have been components of the benefit programs created to address the needs of people with disabilities, old age and retirement issues have not. Thus disability groups will be entering a new political arena in the coming years. For some, the territory will not be entirely unfamiliar.

Over the years, political and demographic pressures have led to the consolidation and integration of aging and disability programs in some states. Other groups, such as the Citizens Consortium on Disabilities, have been active in long-term care politics for some time. The need to work together on shaping the future of aging policy is unprecedented. Previous efforts have been made to promote a common agenda, but not always successfully. As the general trend toward an aging population moves forward, parallel with the population trend toward aging with disabilities, both sides will be seeking benefits for their constituencies. Historically, the two sides have had limited political collaboration. Recent policy developments, however, suggest that they have similar issues at stake and should renew efforts to build political alliances.

Disability Issues in Aging Health Care Policy

In discussing what aging health care policy might mean for people aging with disabilities, we need a broad definition—one that includes health and medical services and insurance disability coverage. These features come under the auspices of large federal programs—Medicare and Medicaid—the major health care programs serving older people and low-income individuals, including younger people with disabilities (Torres-Gil and Villa 2000).[1] Passed in 1965, the two programs constitute a de facto national health care system for those groups. Medicare covers everyone sixty-five and older and the spouses or former spouses of eligible people as well as those who have been receiving Social Security disability benefits for at least two years or have end-stage renal (kidney) disease. Medicaid is a means-tested program that provides health insurance to people with low incomes who meet certain eligibility requirements. The magnitude of the Medicare and Medicaid programs is significant.

By 1996, Medicare provided health insurance for 38 million people who were older or disabled (and it grew to 40 million by 2001), and Medicaid provided coverage for 36 million low-income people (Pear 1998). That year, Medicare and Medicaid accounted for one-third of national health spending, representing the second largest portion of the federal budget ($351 billion) and making those programs, along with Social Security, an extraordinarily visible segment of national social policy. Over the past three decades, there has been an increased trend for Medicare and Medicaid to consume a larger portion of federal spending. In 1971, Social Security and Medicare together accounted for 22 percent of the budget. By 2000 it had increased to 35 percent, and the Congressional Budget Office expects federal spending for the elderly population to reach 43 percent by 2010 (Rauch 2000). Proposals to restructure these programs, then, have become a matter of great national importance.

One of the more complex and problematic features of aging health care policy is "long-term care." This term refers to an array of institutional-, home-, and community-based services, including nursing homes, respite care, adult day care, hospice services, case management, transportation and housing assistance, homemaker and chore services, and personal companions.

Long-term care has long been the purview of aging advocates, and Medicaid has become their de facto long-term care program. In 1995, Medicaid spent $50 billion on long-term care services, with $40 billion of that amount going to nursing homes and institutional care—that is, intermediate care facilities for the mentally retarded—while only $9.9 billion went for home- and community-based care (Stone 2000). However, the future of Medicaid as the main long-term care program for older adults is in question.

At present there is no consensus within Congress or state legislatures about the absence of publicly funded long-term care. Medicare pays for time-limited skilled nursing care and home health care if medically prescribed. Medicaid, through waiver authority, will cover home- and community-based services and community-supported living arrangements. These programs provide important assistance to older people and younger individuals with disabilities. But they serve a relatively small number of those in need of long-term care. The bulk of long-term care services for older adults in the United States is provided informally by family members and friends. In 1994 more than 7 million Americans, mostly family members, provided 120 million hours of unpaid care to elders with functional disabilities living in the community (Stone 2000).

The future of informal long-term care support looks bleak. Public financing and expansion of home- and community-based programs are low on the political agenda of Congress and most state legislatures. There is a shortage of paid long-term care staff, including nurses, aides, and in-home health workers, to meet the rising need for long-term care among the ever-growing aging population. And there is a shortage of time and resources available for family and friends to lend support to older adults in need of assistance. With the parallel development of rising employment, smaller families, more women working full time, and families living farther apart, the ability to provide informal care has decreased. And there is a shrinking pool of potential caregivers (see fig. 14.2).

How federal health care programs for older adults fit into the larger federal spending picture and the practical ramifications of how long-term care programs are structured are important to people aging with disabilities. Historically, any discussions of proposals to expand, alter, or restrict Medicare and Medicaid have generated tremendous political objections from their affected constituencies. Older people are deeply troubled that eligibility criteria, financing and insurance systems, benefits and reimbursements, and access to

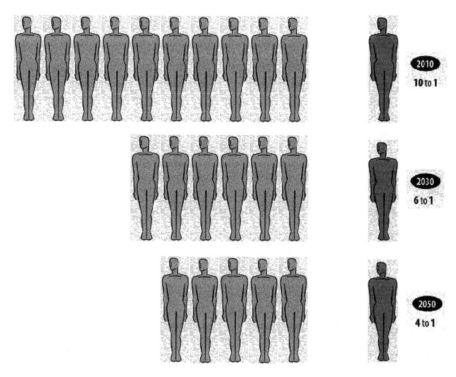

Figure 14.2. The shrinking pool of potential caregivers. In 1990 the ratio of the population in the average caregiving age range, ages fifty to sixty-four, to the population age eighty-five and older was eleven to one. By 2050 there will be only four potential caregivers for every elderly person. *Source:* Data from U.S. Bureau of the Census (1992, 1993).

medical care may be altered or reduced. People aging with disabilities will increasingly be worried about those issues, but perhaps in additional ways. Many people depend on Medicare and Medicaid benefits coverage and will be affected if reimbursements, benefits, and access to care (including greater use of managed care) are changed. Yet their broader perspective on what they need as they age with disabilities may not be part of the debate about reforming Medicare and Medicaid or changing Social Security. Their concerns about housing, transportation, and retirement and their preferences for independence and control of professional and medical care may not be factored into the political debates about entitlement reform and responding to the aging of the Baby Boom cohort. How they enter the aging health care debate and their responses to recent shifts in contemporary thoughts about aging health care policy will be a measure of their political interests and significance as players in the politics of aging.

Contemporary Health Care Policy

The politics and policies of aging health care today revolve around the twin concerns of demographics and budget. The pending mass retirement of Baby Boomers has raised the question whether we can afford entitlement programs for 75 million Baby Boomers. Responses have generated a variety of proposals to modify existing public policies and to rethink government's role vis-à-vis an older society. Prominent themes dominating aging health care policy debates include personal responsibility, financial planning, and saving for retirement. Contemporary political thought on the part of both government officials and the general public is leaning toward less reliance on the social (aging) safety net and more individual responsibility (as witnessed in welfare reform). This philosophical orientation may change, of course, given political demands and pressures by individuals demonstrating political influence. But at present this is the political and ideological atmosphere in which aging policy reforms will be made.

The demographic trends that frame today's policy debates about aging health care are long-standing issues. Until recently, Congress and the executive branch regularly grappled with federal deficits and the projected insolvencies of Social Security and Medicare. Fiscal concerns led to proposals for scaling back benefits and increasing eligibility requirements for many old-age programs. However, with the recent increase in projected federal surpluses, the political mood shifted toward new proposals advocating the expansion of health care, most notably prescription drug coverage. The evaporating surplus, however, has renewed support for the concept of privatization.

Privatization is the latest and perhaps most important political concept to enter aging politics in decades. The idea means changing the fundamental premise of federal programs such as Social Security and Medicare and moving toward the philosophical goal of individual responsibility. In its simplest form, privatization means relying on market forces, giving individuals more choice, and requiring beneficiaries to take on a greater risk for their financial and health security. Privatization first came into mainstream aging politics in association with Social Security. Within the Social Security program, privatization refers to the creation of individual retirement accounts, whereby those who pay taxes into Social Security would place a portion of those taxes in individual accounts that they would control and invest in whatever manner they chose, including the stock market (Rich 2001). This program modification presumably would give them the chance to obtain a higher rate of return from individual investments and a greater stake in the use of their tax contributions, while engendering more support by taxpayers, especially younger cohorts, in maintaining Social Security. Opponents of privatization suggest that it would eliminate the fundamental "social insurance" principles of Social Security, whereby all taxpayers contribute and people receive benefits depending on their actual circumstances. They also argue that it would permanently modify the social contract between generations. Their more practical fear is that economic downturns would increase individual risk and yield less retirement savings, not more. Additionally, opponents are worried about the high transition costs the federal treasury will incur in drawing out the funds for individual retirement accounts in a pay-as-you-go system, where revenues are used to cover current beneficiaries.

Fears about privatization extend to aging health policy as well, where reformers are considering a restructuring of Medicare and Medicaid based on those principles. Within Medicare and Medicaid, privatization would involve creating individual medical vouchers and a greater use of managed care. Currently, Medicare entitles individuals to receive Part A and Part B coverage, after paying deductibles and premiums, regardless of the cost to the federal government. With privatization, individuals would receive vouchers for a predetermined amount of money and would buy health insurance coverage on the open market. Individuals could choose to keep that amount and not buy insurance. Or if they bought an insurance policy that costs more than the government voucher amount, they would pay the difference out of pocket. This latter issue raises a red flag for many aging advocates. Their concern is that people with preexisting medical conditions or with costly medical needs would have a more difficult time obtaining adequate health insurance on the open market or would have to pay more out-of-pocket costs. In some policy scenarios, individuals would be able to stay in a Medicare fee-for-service system, but that would not guarantee that costs to the individuals with substantial health or long-term care needs would be adequately covered.

A similar plan is developing for prescription drug coverage that would target low-income elders with some sort of subsidy program. Prescription drugs are not covered by Medicare, yet older adults account for over one-third of the nation's total drug expenditures (Fuchs et al. 2000). While two-thirds of beneficiaries have some form of drug coverage to supplement their Medicare, one-third lack coverage and must pay for their medications out of pocket.

For many people who are aging with disabilities, the implications of individual responsibility are not new. It is a key component of the independent living philosophy that has served as a cornerstone of disability-related home and personal assistance programs for the past three decades. What is new and different is the role of the government in the equation and the role it plays in aging health policy. Since the inception of Medicare and Medicaid, there have been entitlement programs mandating acute and long-term care. A move toward privatization would mean that consumers would have to shoulder a larger share of the added costs and would have to compete on the open market for insurance coverage. In a system where more responsibility is put on individuals for managing health care services and costs, people who have substantial health and long-term care needs (e.g., multiple long-term chronic conditions, physical impairments, and secondary conditions complicated by aging) will carry more of the burden for locating and paying for adequate care. The winners of the privatization of aging health care will be people who easily "fit into" the system. People aging with disabilities historically have had difficulty finding appropriate medical care providers and affording health insurance that addresses their complex needs. This is particularly true for people with severe long-term physical impairments who have trouble obtaining and maintaining employment and have limited financial resources. For those individuals, significant changes in Medicare or Medicaid could cost them more than others in their age groups who do not share their levels of disability. Thus it behooves adults aging with disabilities to become alert to the aging policy changes that are currently on deck and to understand the implications for them. Although they may enter old age with a different physical status than their generational counterparts, the issues that concern all older adults will be the same: access to adequate and affordable health insurance and health care; sufficient health care and home care providers, including medical professionals and informal caregivers; and reasonable costs of needed services. Given this potential state of public affairs, what does this mean for disability issues in aging politics? What are other concerns that people aging with disabilities ought to have as aging and disability come together?

Disability Issues in Aging Politics

Historically, a firm line has been drawn between aging programs and services and disability programs and services. That line is age sixty-five in most cases, and age sixty-two in others. What we are seeing in case of aging with a disability is that age is a poor indicator of the service needs of people with disabilities. Age sixty-five may signal retirement for individuals who are physically able to work until that age. For those aging with disabilities, retirement may begin ten to fifteen years earlier, depending on their physical condition and health. In this scenario, the common retirement-age issues—such as access to medical insurance, levels of insurance coverage, affordable housing, public transportation, the need for accessible environments and assistive equipment, caregiving, and economic stability—begin much earlier and take on a different dimension. That is, people aging with disabilities may be too young to receive services that may provide support in those areas.

What this means for them is a "premature aging" occurring before they are eligible for aged-based entitlement programs. Thus they find that the old-age criteria currently in use are irrelevant. The irony is that while they may enjoy added longevity, age-based public policies do not account for the effects of premature aging. While many people aging with disabilities may live longer, because of their health problems they may be forced into early retirement, even before age sixty-two, the age of partial benefits in Social Security. This poses various dilemmas: they may be entitled to Disability Insurance coverage, but that may prove inadequate. If they have saved for retirement under 401(k) or Keogh plans, they may be forced to dip into those funds prematurely, thus facing tax penalties and loss of investment income in a market downturn. As shown in figure 14.1, many more people will need help with ADLs. In a free market environment, chronic conditions will limit access to private insurance and force reliance on public insurance. As figure 14.3 illustrates, working-age disabled adults are far less likely than others to obtain private health insurance coverage, particularly if they are unable to work. And the more disabled people are, the less their chances of securing private insurance, while their dependency on public insurance (Medicare and Medicaid) increases. Along with those concerns are the equally pressing issues of housing and transportation and the ability to maintain independence and remain part of the community. The debates over entitlement programs, particularly pro-

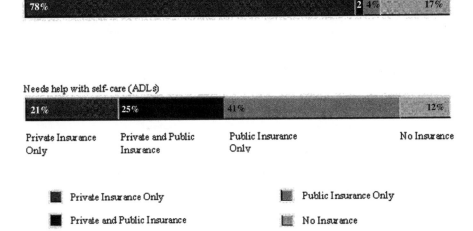

Figure 14.3. Chronic conditions limit access to private insurance and force reliance on public insurance. *Source:* LaPlante 1993, table D, p. 18.

grams for older people, do not account for the concerns facing people aging with disabilities.

Historically, aging policies have been flexible in accepting and supporting programmatic and service changes that produce cost savings, better serve particular geographic regions of the country (e.g., rural, inner-city), or more effectively address consumer needs. What has remained inflexible are the age requirements for eligibility. For that reason, policy analysts increasingly are proposing that age-based programs move from age to some measures of functional disability (e.g., ADLs) as criteria for programs traditionally designed for older people, thus opening them up to those with disabilities who are younger than current age limits. This policy prescription, however, is not yet part of the larger debates over reform of Social Security, Medicare, Medicaid, or other programs such as the Older Americans Act. In the coming years, public policy must begin to address some of the tough questions that have as yet gone unanswered. Will people aging with disabilities gain access to aging services at a younger age? If so, what will be the standards for eligibility? Will aging programs evolve to embrace aging with a disability, modifying their mandates or more closely matching those of current disability programs? Younger people aging with disabilities have much at stake in how these questions are answered.

If we were writing prescriptions for action, we would suggest that the following public policy issues be addressed within the next few years:

1. What are the retirement needs of adults aging with disabilities? If individuals retire from full-time work at age fifty to fifty-five, as seems likely, what type of financial mechanisms are in place, or should be in place, to support their economic survival?
2. How are the health and health insurance needs of adults aging with disabilities being addressed? How can they pay for the services they need? What types of reimbursements will they receive for services, personal assistance, and assistive technology to help them live independently? How does lack of health insurance contribute to their physical health, emotional well-being, and financial stability in retirement?
3. What are the housing and transportation needs for adults aging with disabilities? Is there enough accessible housing stock in the private and public sectors? Are transportation costs subsidized or reimbursed at adequate rates?
4. How effectively are the health and wellness needs of adults aging with disabilities being addressed in the medical establishment and the local community? How adequately are people with disabilities reimbursed by their health insurers, including Medicare and Medicaid, for the costs of living long-term with disabilities?

These and other concerns ought to be part of the public dialogue for a society witnessing greater numbers of people moving into old age with some level of disability.

The Future of Health Care Policy and the Search for Common Ground

This chapter has examined the interrelation of health care policy with the aging population and suggested that people aging with disabilities have a stake in the public policy decisions affecting health and long-term care programs and in the debates about entitlement reforms. Under such a premise, it is reasonable to assume that advocacy groups representing people with disabilities and older people should build alliances to advocate for their current and future needs. How successful this will be remains to be seen. Traditionally, there have been differences in their political agendas that have precluded collaboration, and the lack of a common agenda has kept them apart. Older people and their advocacy groups have an enviable record of influencing the passage of laws, benefits, and programs that serve them well. Much of their organizing effort is directed at holding on to the vast array of public policies such as Medicare, Medicaid, Social Security, the Older Americans Act, and the Supplemental Security Income program (SSI). Much of their political effort is focused on the national and federal scene. Disability organizations have had equal success in their own arenas, helping to enact significant education, employment, and civil rights legislation. Unlike aging organizations, disability groups have developed a powerful grassroots network of activists who work at the local, state, and national levels. Their success is built on people with disabilities, and parents of children with disabilities, advocating on their own behalf. Together these groups could represent a powerful force in aging politics and give a significant voice to adults aging with disabilities in the coming policy debates. Whether they can actually do so remains to be seen.

However, the need for people aging with disabilities to take note of the politics of aging is pressing. With the aging of the population, issues of caregiving and long-term care, health care coverage, and Medicare and Medicaid solvency will be overriding concerns of public and elected officials. Those issues may be influenced by the electoral and interest-group power of older people. We argue that, to ensure that their voices are heard, members of the disabled community must become involved in aging politics, since they have a stake in proposals to privatize Medicare and Medicaid and share concerns about the funding of long-term care and the shortage of caregivers in our aging society.

NOTE

1. If you are disabled, you may be eligible for Medicare before age sixty-five. You must have been entitled to disability benefits from the Social Security program (not SSI, Supplemental Security Income) for two years as a worker, surviving spouse, or adult child of a retired, disabled, or deceased worker. You need not apply for Medicare in the event you were entitled; enrollment is automatic. Special provisions apply to people with end-stage renal

disease (kidney failure) who require dialysis or a transplant and are under sixty-five. In such cases, you are eligible for Part A at any age if you are a worker insured by Social Security or Railroad Retirement or are the spouse or dependent child of an insured worker (including a survivor of a deceased insured worker). See the handbook *Medicare, 2001: What You Need to Know about Medicare in Simple, Practical Terms,* written by J. Robert Treanor, Manager, Social Security Information Services (Louisville, Ky.: William M. Mercer, 2000).

REFERENCES

Campbell, M., Sheets, D., and Strong, P. 1999. Secondary health conditions among middle-aged individuals with chronic physical disabilities: Implications for unmet needs for services. *Assistive Technology* 11 (2): 105–22.

Day, J. C. 1990. *What older Americans think: Interest groups and aging policy.* Princeton, N.J.: Princeton University Press.

Day, J. C. 1993. Population projections of the United States by age, sex, race, and Hispanic origin, 1995-2050. In *U.S. Bureau of the Census, Current Population Reports,* 25–1130. Washington, D.C.: U.S. Government Printing Office.

Fuchs, B., James, J., Mays, J., and Schaefer, M. 2000. Analyzing options to cover prescription drugs for Medicare beneficiaries. *Kaiser Family Foundation,* August.

LaPlante, M. P. 1993. Disability, health insurance coverage, and utilization of acute health services in the United States. In *Disability Statistics Report,* no. 4. Washington, D.C.: National Institute on Disability and Rehabilitation Research.

Pear, R. 1998. Spending on health grew slowly in 1996. *New York Times,* National Edition, A9.

Rauch, J. 2000. The agony of choosing between Bush and Gore. *National Journal,* 3468–69.

Rich, S. 2001. A tiny middle ground in the Social Security privatization debate. *National Journal,* 33.

Robert Wood Johnson Foundation. 1996. *Chronic care in America: A 21st century challenge.* Princeton, N.J.: Robert Wood Johnson Foundation.

Sasma, G. P., Patrick, C. H., and Feusser, J. R. 1993. Long-term survival of veterans with traumatic spinal cord injury. *Archives of Neurology* 50:909–14.

Stone, R. 2000. *Long-term care for the elderly with disabilities: Current policy, emerging trends, and implications for the twenty-first century.* New York: Milbank Memorial Fund.

Tompkins, L. 1997. Polio survivors: Preliminary data from the polio supplement of the 1994-95 National Health Interview Survey. *Proceedings of the Seventh International Post-Polio and Independent Living Conference.* St. Louis: Gazette International Networking Institute.

Torres-Gil, F. 1992. *The new aging: Politics and change in America.* Westport, Conn.: Auburn House.

Torres-Gil, F., and Villa, V. 2000. Social policy and the elderly. In *The handbook of social policy,* ed. J. Midgley, M. Tracy, and M. Livermore, 209–20. Thousand Oaks, Calif.: Sage.

U.S. Bureau of the Census. 1990. *Table DP-1. Profile of general demographic characteristics for the United States.* Washington, D.C.: U.S. Government Printing Office.

U.S. Bureau of the Census. 1992. Population projections of the United States, by age, sex, and Hispanic origin, 1992-2050. In *Current population reports*, 25–1092. Washington, D.C.: U.S. Government Printing Office.

U.S. Bureau of the Census. 1993. *Statistical abstract of the United States, 1993.* Washington, D.C.: U.S. Government Printing Office.

U.S. Bureau of the Census. 1996. 65+ in the United States. *Current population reports special studies.* 23-190. Washington, D.C.: Government Printing Office.

U.S. Bureau of the Census. 2000. *Table DP-1: Profile of general demographic characteristics for the United States.* Washington, D.C.: U.S. Government Printing Office.

15

The Health Care Partnership—
Barriers to Care

Part 1: The Provider's Viewpoint

Terry Winkler, M.D.

Obtaining optimal, or even basic, health care in today's medical environment is difficult even for the most sophisticated person. For the person who has a disability, there are myriad other factors that make obtaining health care nearly impossible. These factors include provider attitudes, the lack of disability training in medical school and allied health educational programs, the medical provider system (the "medical model"), funding sources, social expectations of both the provider and the person with a disability, and political philosophies. Add to these the confounding array of medical "alphabet soup"—preferred provider organizations (PPOs), health maintenance organizations (HMOs), diagnosis-related grouping (DRG), current procedural terminology (CPT), professional review organizations (PROs), preferred provider plan (PPPs), length of stay (LOS), quality assurance (QA), utilization reviews (URs), case management (CM), Health Care Finance Administration (HCFA), managed care organizations (MCOs), primary care providers (PCPs)—and the net effect is limited access to services for everyone, but especially for people who are disabled.

Barriers in the System Owing to Cost Containment

Health care costs have grown exponentially since the development of third-party payer systems (Medicare, Medicaid, private insurance) and newer and more expensive technologies. As the proportion of funds spent on health care approached and passed 10 percent of the gross national product in the 1970s, numerous methods were developed by both the government and private industry to try to limit these soaring costs. One approach involved limiting the use of high-technology measures by restricting access to medical specialists who would be more likely to order them. When transplants, MRIs, artificial hearts, and other expensive procedures became available, the health care system was forced to focus attention for the first time on the concept of "allocation of valuable medical resources." The idea was proposed that valuable medical resources (dollars spent on health care) should be used only to purchase the most important or reasonable services. John Callan (1993) stated that "the traditional right of a physician to make independent decisions about a patient has been replaced by multidisciplinary teams and consensus judgements." Donald Light (1992) coined the phrase "inverse coverage law" to describe this point: the more individuals need expensive services, the less likely they are to get them. This means that people who have the most severe medical problems, such as those with disabilities, are least likely to get what they need. Additionally, the larger the health care system, the more likely that it will unduly restrict services. This naturally extends to people with severe disabilities, who often have more complicated problems. Hagglund, Clay, and Acuff (1998) reported that most managed care organizations have no experience in providing comprehensive, coordinated services to people with disabilities, nor do they have a philosophy about serving this population. For example, DeJong (2000) reported that 5 million working-age people with disabilities were left out of the recent debate on Medicare prescription benefits, even though prescription drugs costs are thirty times higher for them than for nondisabled people.

Physicians' attitudes about disability also present a sizable barrier to consumers. These attitudes are often formed during medical training. For example, while I was in medical school, the chair of surgery discussed these disability-related cost issues with us future physicians with the intent of shaping our prescription practices. "Dr. McSurgeon" stood before the first-year medical class, arms folded, looking over his wire-rimmed glasses as smoke from his pipe curiously circled his head, wearing a long white lab coat (our lab coats were half-length, signifying our lower status in the system). In a booming General Patton voice, he pronounced, "The cost of immortality is infinite!" With charts and graphs, he proceeded to illustrate this to his naive medical army.

His well-taken point was that as people get older, they have more illnesses and experience increasing rates of disability, and there is no limit to the cost of helping them live longer. To illustrate his point, Dr. McSurgeon gave case examples. "If a fifty-year-old man comes to the ER with a suspected heart attack, do you try to save him?" The students' response overwhelmingly was yes. "Now," he said, suppose he is sixty years old, with hypertension and diabetes?" The students' response was, yes. Dr. McSurgeon continued, "He is sixty years old, has hypertension, diabetes, a left below-the-knee amputation, and limited eyesight, is single and unemployed, and smokes two packs of cigarettes and drinks a fifth of whiskey every day. To treat him means that he will likely be in the ICU and on a ventilator for three months before we can wean him." Slowly walking around the room, looking deeply into the medical students' eyes, he added, "The medical resources that you are going to use on him will prevent you from providing vaccine to two hundred children in the pediatric clinic next week. Do you save him?" There was a long silence in the room. Finally came a couple of yeses out of the hundred-plus medical students. In just thirty minutes, Dr. McSurgeon has convinced his students that they will face situations that mix their personal biases, political beliefs, religious beliefs, value judgments, and budget-balancing ideals with medical decision making. The point is that owing to similar attitudes toward people with disabilities, especially severe disabilities, this process, or some form of this process, has a high likelihood of playing itself out each time a person with a disability presents himself or herself to a health care provider in the United States.

A fifty-two-year-old man with tetraplegia (Gene) came to the university teaching hospital with severe chest pain. He was having a myocardial infarction. He worked full time as a disability case manager, lived independently in the community, provided full-time employment to another disabled person, was independent in community mobility with his own vehicle, had a master's degree in counseling, and had no medical conditions except for his spinal cord injury. Gene's personal care attendant called me late in the evening, frightened at what was going to happen, to tell me Gene was in the hospital with a heart attack. I dressed and went to the hospital. As a resident physician at the hospital system, it was easy for me to learn that Gene was in the cardiac catheterization unit. When I came into the room, three physicians stood with their hands folded, watching heart monitors. Gene was ashy gray, in agonal respiration, but he had a decent heartbeat and was maintaining a blood pressure. The treating physicians, who had never met him before, seemed to be hesitating about what to do. I explained to them that until that day, Gene had been very healthy, was fully employed, was a source of employment for others, and was an extremely valuable member and leader of Arkansas's disability community. The three physicians looked at me and at each other and then intubated Gene, putting him on a ventilator. Within minutes the near death, ashy gray color gave way to a healthy, visibly pink appearance. Over the next several weeks, Gene not only survived but also was discharged to his home, where he continued to live and function independently in the community for eight more years before dying from a second myocardial infarction.

If Gene had not had tetraplegia, the physicians' response that day might have been different. He might have been intubated within minutes of arriving in the heart catheterization lab, and he would not have required an advocate to plead for basic, routine health care that is given to able-bodied people in the same system. Such life-and-death scenarios are played out daily in U.S. hospitals.

The health care system is generally experiencing a shrinkage in dollars owing to cutbacks in funding by third-party payers. A special case is Medicaid, the government program of health coverage for low-income people. Medicaid also covers many people with disabilities because of their high unemployment rate. Many of them are therefore viewed by health providers as "low pays or no pays." For example, in the state of Missouri, a fifteen- to thirty-minute follow-up visit (LPT code 99213 and 99214) with a person who has Medicaid will produce a gross income for the physician of $24 to $25.50,equal to $55 to $65 an hour. Subtract from this office overhead for a typical office, which is calculated at $150 or more an hour. Each hour spent on follow-up care for patients who have Medicaid not only produces no income but brings a loss of $90 to $100. In an era when health care providers' personal incomes are shrinking, many elect not to further jeopardize their financial stability by seeing the "low pays" (people with disabilities). The physical or occupational therapist practicing within a health delivery system or independently may experience similar financial pressures.

Another barrier to services for people who have disabilities is providers' noncompliance with the Americans with Disabilities Act (ADA), even though it has now been more than a decade since it was enacted. Most health care clinics and physicians' offices still do not meet accessibility requirements of

ADA. Exam rooms are small and examination tables are high, severely limiting physical access to services. In an effort to remain financially solvent, health care institutions and physicians' offices have reduced staffing, further restricting the availability of personnel to assist people with disabilities. Gans, Mann, and Becker (1993) reported that many health care providers have inaccessible offices as well as lack of appropriate equipment and supplies needed to examine and treat those with mobility impairments.

Payment policies and the desire to reduce medical expenditures further complicate care for people with disabilities. Studies have shown that the payer source (fee-for-service versus managed care) affects the outcome after the acute onset of disability (Retchin et al. 1997). A study of people with spinal cord injury (SCI) ascertained that having managed Medicare, Medicaid, or a private managed care HMO plan increased the risk of mortality by 50 percent compared with having fee-for-service private insurance (DeVivo, Krause, and Lammertse 1999).

Further, people with disabilities, by virtue of their primary impairments, are at risk for developing numerous secondary complications or new medical problems that require careful screening and periodic evaluation. Seekins, Clay, and Ravesloot (1994) surveyed a population of adults with physical disabilities and reported an average of thirteen secondary problems a year, such as pressure sores, urinary tract infections, poor nutrition, pain, and depression. In addition, people with disabilities are less well equipped to maintain their health or prevent complications. Even fee-for-service third-party payers, including Medicare, will not cover the cost of "routine screening procedures," thereby increasing the risk that the person with a disability will experience predictable complications, leading to increased mortality and morbidity.

Pressures, both governmental and private, have resulted in shorter and shorter hospital stays. This can have both positive and negative consequences, but Morrison (1999) reported that length of stay has decreased to a point that it is now detrimental to patient outcome and causes increased medical complications. The net result is that people with disabilities, because they have more health care problems, are sent home earlier and "sicker." Finally, many third-party payers will not cover the cost of intensive medical rehabilitation at a center of excellence. Instead, they opt for subacute rehabilitation programs in long-term care facilities, which reduce costs by using a lower level of skill or personnel or less intense services.

To complicate matters further, health care delivery systems have developed a procedure that threatens to undermine the entire premise that health care has been based on throughout the centuries. For thousands of years, society in general and patients in particular have assumed that health care providers acted in the best interests of the patient. A new procedure that changes this centuries-old-tradition is the widespread use of primary care physicians (PCPs), to function as "gatekeepers." Many of these doctors even have financial interests that are directly opposed and contradictory to providing reasonable and prudent medical care. Some organizations actually pay a bonus to the PCPs if they are able to keep the use of services below a certain level or if they limit access to specialty physicians to a certain level. Other contracts function by terminating the PCP as a provider in the organization if services are not limited to a specified amount. These agreements can serve as formidable roadblocks to the disabled consumer who is trying to gain access to specialty services. Many physicians who refuse to participate in such agreements believe they violate a sacred trust between physicians or health care providers and patients. The role of the gatekeeper in health care can severely undermine this trust, especially for the person with a disability. Barriers to health care may be made worse by managed care's financial and risk-sharing arrangements that create incentives for providers to achieve cost savings by limiting access.

Barriers Presented by the Person with a Disability

In addition to problems in the health care system, third-party payer systems, and health care providers, the person with a disability often presents a set of problems and issues that become roadblocks to receiving adequate health care. People with disabilities often feels physically vulnerable and, if newly disabled, perhaps helpless and dependent. This can lead to a state of physical, emotional, and mental inertia, in turn resulting in excess disability or handicap. Some individuals who are disabled have an ongoing sense of shame or guilt concerning their disabilities. They may be ashamed or embarrassed about their physical limitations or perhaps feel guilty that they contributed to the onset of their disability (e.g., driving without a seat belt, drinking excessively). Many have a low sense of self-esteem and may erroneously believe the things society thinks about them. Irving Zola (1987) said that the history of disability in America has been so full of discrimination that the experience of being disabled is often described as the "management of stigma." If one could not garner sufficient personal and economic resources to overcome "it" (the stigma), then the next best thing was try to "pass" as nondisabled. People with disabilities may feel isolated or alone, as if they are the only ones who have dealt with "their issues." Depending on their level of adjustment since the onset of the disability, individuals may experience depression, denial, or anger, which can be projected onto the health care professional.

A number of consumer groups composed of and representing the disability community have accurately focused on failures of the "medical model" to meet their health care needs. Some organizations such as the American Disabled Attendant Programs Today (ADAPT), which has a national membership, see the medical model and the health care delivery system as the enemy that prevents people with disabilities from receiving reasonable community-based, consumer-controlled services. Some members of such organizations consider health care providers "the white coats" and view them as enemies of the disability community. Community-based, consumer-controlled service is a reasonable goal, and if implemented properly, would likely have an overall positive effect on the delivery of health care services. However, some members of the disability community, through their actions, alienate themselves from the health care system, which results in a poor level of care. Some people with disabilities have a great deal of knowledge concerning their disabilities and the potential complications, and are good at helping the health care team provide the required services. Many members of the disability community, however, do not have even basic knowledge about their disabilities, their health care needs, or health maintenance issues. This can be a severe detriment to obtaining reasonable and prudent health care. The more knowledgeable individuals are about their disabilities and their health care needs, the more likely they are to be successful at getting those needs met.

Consumers' lack of understanding and lack of information regarding their health care needs frequently lead to noncompliance, such as in taking medication correctly or following up with appointments or tests. The medical literature is full of horror stories about what happens when individuals with disabilities are noncompliant with their health care. Even in the most ideal circumstances, secondary conditions are likely to develop for the person with a disability. With noncompliant behavior, the rates and severity of secondary complications markedly increase. As the complications mount for any one person, so will complications in trying to meet that individual's health care needs. It is common for a health care provider to see people with disabilities in the hospital with severe secondary complications after they have not been seen at follow-up appointments in the office for several years. Frequently a family member will tell physicians that the patients are angry at something they perceived was done or not done, perhaps angry at an office employee, or even the bus driver who brought them to the appointment, and decided not to return to the office, "to show how dissatisfied they were." Consumers may view themselves as "victims" and feel helpless to change their lives for the better. They may feel that the onset of the disability has set in motion a progressively deteriorating course, which they cannot alter in any way. Lammertse (2001) reported that a significant component of implementing prevention strategies is encouraging consumers to "take ownership" of the process of leading a healthy life.

Strategies to Improve Health Care Delivery for People Who Have Disabilities

It is incumbent on the health care provider and the delivery system to find effective ways to improve services for people with disabilities. As the first section of this chapter noted, the bulk of the problems experienced by those with disabilities are a direct result of the health care system's problems and organization structure. It is important that medical and therapy providers find creative and positive ways to improve the services they provide.

The nature of disability itself, its functional limitations, and the high risk of secondary complications mandate that health service providers schedule longer appointment times when providing services. Providers cannot stand at the entrance to the exam room, holding on to the doorknob, ready to make an exit within minutes. They must be willing to listen carefully to the complaints described. Effective communication will be enhanced if the provider sits in a chair making direct contact rather than standing and lording it over the patient in a paternalistic posture. An old axiom in medicine is "Listen to the patients; they will tell you what is wrong with them." Nowhere in medicine is this more applicable than when interacting with the person who has a disability.

The therapist must make every attempt to offer services in the least restricted environment possible. For example, if the procedure room in the clinic is larger and more accessible to a wheelchair user than the typical exam room, then a break in the ordinary routine is in order to accommodate that person's needs.

Recognizing the level of knowledge or education consumers have about their own disabilities and their state of psychological and emotional adjustment to the disability are two very important considerations. If they know little about their condition and its possible secondary complications, then providing extra time for education, for providing patient resources and community resource information, will help raise their level of awareness, improving their ability to obtain health care services. People with low self-esteem or a decreased sense of self-worth will benefit from positive feedback from health care providers, from psychological counseling, and from interaction with peer support groups.

Careful documentation of the patient's specific diagnosis, level of health, and most important, functional problems will make it easier to provide services to the individual in that health care system as well as other health care systems and justify the needed services to third-party payers.

Finally, therapist-providers must be willing to advocate for the fair, reasonable, and prudent needs of people with disabilities within the health care delivery system they work in, with third-party payers, and also with policymakers and politicians.

Consumers also have an important role in improving the health care services they receive. First, people with disabilities must become "experts" in their particular disabilities and unique health care needs. In many rural areas, health care providers have little or no experience in working with those individuals' particular disabilities. The level and quality of care received can be greatly enhanced if consumers are informed enough to help educate the local health care providers.

Making earnest attempts to reduce missed appointments or miscommunication will improve provider-consumer relationships. Avoiding noncompliance or the appearance of noncompliance by actively communicating with the health care provider will yield a positive, professional relationship.

Summary

Being aware of the pressures and constraints that limit health care providers' availability or ability to have prolonged interactions is important. To this end, the consumer can best assist the health professional by focusing on the most important issues or topics that need to be dealt with during that visit. When interacting with members of the rehabilitation team, communication and outcomes are enhanced if consumers approach health care problems as functional issues (they should be prepared to talk about their reasons for the visit in terms of functional problems). They should try to address specific problems to the appropriate member of the health care delivery system (not discuss urological problems and complications with the cardiologist or inhibit the interaction with the physical therapist by venting for fifteen minutes of a thirty-minute session about some other member of the health care team or about family issues). It is helpful to consult other people with disabilities, health care referral sources, Internet resources, and independent living centers to identify health care providers in the community who have the necessary expertise or are willing to take the time to provide reasonable and fair services to individuals with a particular disability or issues.

REFERENCES

Callan, J. P., ed. 1993. *The physician, a profession under stress.* Norwalk, Conn.: Appleton-Century-Crofts.

DeJong, G. 2000. Five million working-age Americans with disabilities lost in current debate on Medicare prescription benefits. National Rehabilitation Website. www.nrhrehab.org.

DeVivo, M. Q., Krause, J. S., and Lammertse, D. P. 1999. Recent trends in mortality and causes of death among persons with spinal cord injury. *Archives of Physical Medicine and Rehabilitation* 80:1411–19.

Gans, B., Mann, N., and Becker, B. 1993. Delivery of primary care to the physically challenged. *Archives of Physical Medicine and Rehabilitation* 74:15–19.

Hagglund, K. J., Clay, D. L., and Acuff, M. 1998. Community reintegration for persons with SCI. *Topics in Spinal Cord Injury Rehabilitation* 4 (2): 28–40.

Lammertse, D. P. 2001. Maintaining health long term with spinal cord injury. *Topics in Spinal Cord Injury Rehabilitation* 6 (3): 12.

Light, D. 1992. The practice and ethics of risk-related health care insurance. *Journal of the American Medical Association* 267:2503–8.

Morrison, S. A. 1999. The effect of shorter lengths of stay on functional outcomes of spinal cord injury rehabilitation. *Topics in Spinal Cord Injury* 4 (4): 44–55.

Retchin, S. M., Brown, R. S., Yeh, S.-C. J., Chu, D., and Moreno, L. 1997. Outcomes of stroke patients in Medicare fee-for-service and managed care. *Journal of the American Medical Association* 2:119–24.

Seekins, T., Clay, J., and Ravesloot, C. 1994. A descriptive study of secondary conditions reported by a population of adults with physical disabilities, served by the three independent living centers in a rural state. *Journal of Rehabilitation* 60:47–51.

Zola, I. 1987. *The international disabilities studies* 9:142–43.

16

The Health Care Partnership—
Barriers to Care

Part 2: The Consumer's Viewpoint

June Kailes

This chapter, written from the perspective of the person with a disability, addresses what health care providers can do to bridge what we people with disabilities (PWDs) call the "complaint gap." PWDs' have responsibility for helping to bridge this gap as well, and this subject is thoroughly covered in some of my other publications (Kailes 1995, 1998a, b, 2000, 2001). Here the term "provider" reflects a broad group of people who provide health-related services for people with disabilities. Providers include, but are not limited to, physicians, therapists, and social workers as well as an array of professionals who are specialists in other fields. Most of the complaints from PWDs about the delivery of health services relate to three things: provider's lack of disability knowledge, poor communication, and time limits that providers impose (Kailes 2001).

Lack of Disability Knowledge

Concerning disability knowledge, PWDs have many complaints. These complaints pertain mostly to providers' lack of knowledge about disability, the barriers PWDs encounter in receiving services, and the support needs that go hand in hand with our health care needs. Chief among our complaints is that health care providers are too quick to dismiss our normal health concerns as just extensions of our disabilities. Many focus only on our disabilities and are too quick to attribute our other health problems to them. This leaves many PWDs feeling frustrated, stereotyped, and ignored. Similarly, providers don't take our disabilities into account when giving us advice or prescribing tests, procedures, or medications. And they often make inaccurate assumptions based on stereotypes about disability (e.g., assuming that PWDs have a low quality of life or don't have questions about sexual health).

Disability knowledge extends to advocacy and legal access as well, and PWDs believe that providers don't understand or attend to their legal obligations under the Americans with Disabilities Act and other federal and state accessibility codes. Providers don't understand that when they are unable or unwilling to adapt their techniques to our needs or perform procedures in a way that accommodates people with a variety of disabilities, we fail to receive medical and preventive care equal to that provided to nondisabled people. The changes that are not made include not allowing more time for people who have a speech or cognitive disability to communicate or understand information, not using interpreters for people who are deaf, not having accessible, height-adjustable examination tables, diagnostic equipment, or other important access elements at their offices, not allowing us to have our service animals with us, and not having printed materials in alternative formats (Braille, large print, disks, audio cassette).

Concerning disability support, PWDs believe that providers don't have enough knowledge about community services (housing, in-home help, economic aid) that could help meet some of our critical needs, and they don't understand that this lack of knowledge about support services goes hand in hand with not recognizing that support problems undermine our health.

PWDs also complain that providers don't know how to evaluate our health from a functional viewpoint; instead, they focus almost exclusively on our medical problems. However, what's important to PWDs is how those medical problems affect our daily functioning. Similarly, providers don't understand the issue of age-related changes in our functional abilities. They don't realize that lack of knowledge and understanding about how our disability can change with age is extremely frightening.

Finally, PWDs feel that providers assume that health, wellness, and disability cannot coexist and that they don't work with us to create a holistic program that is disability-sensitive and specific.

In terms of communication, many PWDs, like other people, feel that providers are always in a hurry, don't allow us enough time to discuss all our questions and issues, and don't realize that we feel anxious and pressured by limited time. Some speak so fast that we can't remember what they said, overuse medical terminology, and order a test, procedure, consultation, or medication without explaining why it is needed. But the disability-specific issue that bugs PWDs the most is when providers talk to parents, spouses, personal assistants, caregivers, or children instead of directly to us.

Bridging the Gap

Health care providers can do a lot to reduce these complaints and build a stronger partnerships with PWDs. Encouraging such a partnership means that providers may have to modify their approach to patients on several fronts: as communicators, as teacher-educators, as learners, and as individuals who respect other people's time.

The advice of PWDs is to treat your relationship with your patients as a partnership. This may take some adjustment, but in today's health care environment it works best when providers welcome and cultivate active participation. This means fostering open communication and not feeling threatened if PWDs have read three journal articles related to their health issues and you have read only one. Sometimes PWDs' health status is so precarious that they are strongly motivated to learn everything they can, just to be their own advocates.

Building partnerships means encouraging PWDs to take back control over their lives, control that was taken away under the health care philosophy of bygone years, which stressed that doctors were experts and patients were not. We have a long-suppressed need to speak up about our health concerns. Getting the most out of health care services requires that PWDs be active and vocal in all aspects of their health care. Don't take it personally. It is our health and therefore our right to be involved in every decision. Today's savvy health care consumers take responsibility for their health. This means being a helping to manage their health care and sharing in decision making. As one person put it,

> I finally began to apply to myself what I had been preaching to the disability community in my work: take back your power, become informed, and stand up for yourself. I learned how to use health professionals as consultants rather than as gods. They have knowledge about the "science" of body and psyche, but I am the

only one who is an expert on me. . . . To heal, or become whole, is not the same as being cured. A cure comes from outside of ourselves. Healing is something that occurs within. And being healed may not mean we are cured. It may simply mean that we reach a state of empowerment, self-love and skilled self-care. (Kailes 1998b)

Teach People How to Be Active Health Care Consumers

Given the massive and continuing changes in health care, it is critical that providers not only welcome active, involved consumers but encourage and teach people how to develop and incorporate their own active health care skills and strategies. Active consumers seek providers who will listen; who will involve them fully in health care decisions; and who will learn as much as possible about their conditions. Active consumers view their relationship with providers as a partnership, which means sharing decision making and responsibility for choosing health care options and alternatives, developing effective treatment plans, and using practices that prevent or minimize complications, including using community resources and assistive technology (exhibit 16.1) (Kailes 1998b).

Providers should teach PWDs to avoid such passive health care behaviors as wanting providers to take charge of their health; relying exclusively on professional advice; failing to ask questions; offering information only when asked; adopting an indifferent and fatalistic attitude of "what will be, will be"; failing to think about options; feeling helpless and lost in the health care system; worrying that care will be compromised if they challenge or disagree with a provider; and letting themselves be processed instead of being partners (exhibit 16.2) (Kailes 1998a). Being passive is dangerous to one's health!

In today's health care environment, the old "doctor knows best" attitude is disappearing fast. The popular television image of doctors (Dr. Kildare, Ben Casey, Marcus Welby) is history. The physician who always has ample time for patients and never hesitates to advocate on their behalf is far from today's health care reality. We must learn how to be effective advocates ourselves or we may have to make do with less than optimal care and sometimes without essential care.

To get the attention and the quality of health care they want, people with disabilities have to do a lot more work than in the past. It is difficult to find full-service health care without working at it and playing an active role. It's like getting gas these days; it's hard to get someone to pump it for you, clean

Exhibit 16.1. Characteristics of active consumers

- Seek providers who will listen
- Seek providers who will involve them fully in decisions
- Learn as much as possible about their own health conditions and continually seek updated information
- Ask question and express their concerns
- Ask providers to explain things in plain language (are not embarrassed to let providers know when they are not communicating clearly or are using highly technical terms)
- View their relationship with providers as a partnership, which includes sharing decision making and responsibility for

  —choosing options and alternatives

  —developing effective intervention and treatment plans
- Use strategies that include

  —understanding their condition

  —adopting practices that prevent or minimize complications

  —using resources and assistive technology
- Learn about their health insurance benefits and requirements for coverage

the windows, and check the oil. You often have to do it yourself. Providers should teach PWDs how to be aware of their baseline physical condition (typical experience) so that they can recognize changes. PWDs should be encouraged to report any significant changes or problems to their providers.

Research confirms that when people are more active in their partnerships with physicians, they have better health. People who communicate well with doctors benefit medically and emotionally. They are physically healthier, recover faster, and are better able to tolerate stress and pain. Take Fred, a wheelchair user who, with help, can stand and walk a few steps. The first time Fred had a physical examination with a new doctor, the doctor never had him get out of his chair. He assumed Fred could not get up, and Fred felt too intimidated to suggest that the doctor do the examination differently. If Fred had explained that he could get out of his chair, he could have received a more comprehensive and complete physical exam (Kailes 1998b).

Providers see people only periodically, sometimes just once or twice a year. PWDs live with their bodies all the time. No one knows more about their

Exhibit 16.2. Characteristics of passive consumers

- Want providers to take charge
- Rely totally on the providers' advice
- Fail to ask questions
- Offer information only when asked
- Adopt an indifferent and fatalistic attitude ("What will be, will be")
- Fail to think about options
- Feel helpless in the health care system
- Worry that their health care will be compromised if they ask questions or challenge or disagree with a provider
- Are "processed" instead of working as partners

daily functioning. In the learner's role, providers should respect PWDs' unique and sometimes superior knowledge of their bodies. Maria's dentist, for example, told her that a certain procedure would not hurt very much and would take only a few minutes, so there was no need for novocaine. However, Maria had good knowledge of her spasticity; she knew that she had a very low threshold for pain and that pain increased her spasms and therefore her ability to stay still in the dental chair (Kailes 1998b).

Most PWDs prefer providers who explain why procedures are being done and explain what is happening during the procedure. This makes everyone more comfortable. When providers are unable to do this while a procedure is ongoing, it should be done beforehand, or they should take a break to explain things along the way (Kailes 1998b).

PWDs should accept their own confidence in their life experience and their common sense so that they are not intimidated by providers who may appear cold and distant. As Eleanor Roosevelt said, "Nobody can make you feel inferior but yourself." Providers can promote PWDs' comfort about speaking up; understand that the personal experience of PWDs is what is important to them and that they don't need professional credentials and degrees to be partners in their own health care.

Every second counts in these times of rushed, fifteen-minute health care appointments. It is critical, and of mutual benefit, to help PWDs learn how to maximize the ever-shrinking visit times. Seventy-five percent of all office visits

Exhibit 16.3. Strategies for a visit with a provider

Make the best use of very limited time during your visit with a provider.

- Give providers relevant information about how your disability affects your health care.
- If you're not asked, provide important information about your condition/disability.
- Ask for an appointment when the provider is less likely to be rushed.
- Ask, at the beginning of the visit, how much time is available, and let the provider know that you have questions.
- Be clear about your priorities and what you want to discuss.
- Create a "questions and concerns list," placing the most important item first. Leave spaces between questions or concerns to take notes. Mail, fax, or e-mail a copy of your list before the visit or give a copy to the receptionist when you arrive.
- Communicate information briefly and succinctly.
- If helpful, work with a support person.
- When seeing new providers, present a current and concise health history that details your condition(s). If possible, mail, fax, or e-mail this information to the provider before the visit. Don't assume it has been read—ask.
- Share useful information about your disability or condition with the provider.
- Take notes or tape record the discussion.
- Request that providers illustrate explanations by using pictures, when needed.
- Take time to think about what you're being told before making an important decision.
- Ask for sources of additional information: books, articles, Web sites, videos, or support groups.
- At the end of a visit, check your understanding by briefly repeating what you heard the provider say.

Source: Be a Savvy Health Care Consumer: Your Life May Depend on It! by June Isaacson Kailes. For more information about this guide, contact the author at jik@pacbell.net or write to Kailes Publications, 6201 Ocean Front Walk, Suite 2, Playa del Rey, CA 90293 or visit http://www.jik.com.

are completed in under fifteen minutes. Providers should teach PWDs to maximize their visit time by reviewing effective visit strategies. With barely enough time to examine and treat patients, how could they possibly have time to teach visit strategies? But teachable moments and short handouts can have a major effect on individual partnerships with providers. A checklist of helpful visit strategies is presented in exhibit 16.3.

Honoring a partnership includes respecting each other's time. PWDs know that patients who require extra time or who have urgent situations can disrupt the schedule. But when people wait longer than fifteen minutes, they have the right to ask how much longer they may have to wait. Providers might suggest that PWDs call just before leaving home to ask if appointments are running on time or are backed up. For example, getting the first appointment of the day or the one right after lunch may reduce the wait.

Additionally, in these times of ever-increasing use of e-mail, providers should consider using this laborsaving, time-saving technology for routine communication to reduce annoying time wasters like telephone tag and telephone hold.

Respect the Patient's Right to Choose or Evaluate Providers

It is important to encourage people's right to choose and evaluate providers. To quote Paul A. Williams, M.D., of the University of Missouri, "Although some patients argue that they are hesitant or are not qualified to check on a doctor, it seems folly not to make an effort to do so, especially when one considers the money that will be spent for the physician's expertise and the fact, also, that one's physical and psychological well-being is going to be entrusted to this person" (Kailes 1998b).

Given the changes in health care, few PWDs have as much flexibility and freedom as we used to in selecting new providers. But in almost all health care plans, people have the right to change their primary care provider. In some geographic areas, however, provider availability may restrict choice. Even though selection is more restricted than it used to be, PWDs still have the right to evaluate providers assigned to them and to request a change. Active consumers take care in choosing new providers as well as evaluating current ones (Kailes 1998b).

For providers, this means allowing time for exploratory, get-acquainted office visits and being open to being interviewed by telephone or answering inquiries from prospective new patients. Be ready to provide a résumé and to answer a variety of questions.

REFERENCES

Kailes, J. K. 1995. Fit to be tried. *Mainstream* 19 (9): 37–46.

Kailes, J. K. 1998a. Be a savvy health care consumer, your life may depend on it. www.jik.com, Kailes publications.

Kailes, J. K. 1998b. Managing your own health care: You've got to be a savvy consumer to make sure your needs are met. *Mainstream* 22(8): 31–34.

Kailes, J. K. 2000. Can disability, chronic conditions, health and wellness coexist? www.jik.com, Kailes publications.

Kailes, J. K. 2001. Health care providers and health care consumers: the complaint gap. www.jik.com, Kailes publications.

Index